A
BROTHERHOOD
OF TYRANTS

A BROTHERHOOD OF TYRANTS

Manic Depression
& Absolute Power

D. Jablow Hershman & Julian Lieb, M.D.

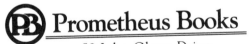

Prometheus Books

59 John Glenn Drive
Amherst, New York 14228-2197

Published 1994 by Prometheus Books

98 97 96 95 94   5 4 3 2 1

Library of Congress Cataloging-in-Publication Data

Hershman, D. Jablow.
    A brotherhood of tyrants : manic depression and absolute power / D. Jablow Hershman and Julian Lieb, M.D.
        p.   cm.
    Includes bibliographical references.
    ISBN 0-87975-888-0 (cloth : acid-free paper)
    1. Napoleon I, Emperor of the French, 1769-1821—Mental health. 2. Hitler, Adolf, 1889-1945—Mental Health. 3. Stalin, Joseph, 1879-1953—Mental health. 4. Manic depressive psychoses—Case studies. 5. Diseases and history. I. Lieb, Julian. II. Title.
D21.3.H47   1994
909.8′092′2—dc20   94-7481
                                                                            CIP

Printed in the United States of America on acid-free paper.

For our families

Contents

Introduction

Power beyond Reason

Although this book examines the private and public lives of Napoleon Bonaparte, Adolf Hitler, and Joseph Stalin, it is neither history nor biography. While we refer to symptoms of manic depression throughout, the book is neither a collection of case histories nor a psychiatric text. Nor does it offer new material about that trio of tyrants or that psychiatric disorder. What it does do is to take the reader into the *terra incognita* of relationships between the strange lives of Napoleon, Hitler, and Stalin and the ferocious, bizarre political systems they established. The exploration of that uncharted territory uncovers manic depression as a hidden cause of dictatorships, war, and genocide.

There is nothing new in the idea that severe psychiatric disorders can profoundly change one's thinking and behavior. Indeed, these changes constitute some of the symptoms of the disease. However, this commonsense idea has rarely been applied to political leaders even when their psychiatric illnesses have been recognized. No one has made a formal comparison of deranged leaders to each other to determine any underlying similarities. As this study will dramatically show, they do act in surprisingly similar ways. These similarities underlie our theory that a specific psychiatric disorder—manic depression—can cause a specific political pathology—tyranny.

Our theory combines familiar facts from history and psychiatry to prove something new in the field of political science. That crossing of intellectual borders will in itself arouse opposition. However, to dismiss this theory before sifting through the evidence is to leave humanity where it has always been—helpless beneath the heels of monsters.

Power and madness are linked together by a psychiatric disorder so variable in its effects that it condemns some people to twilight lives in psychiatric hospitals

9

while propelling others to every imaginable kind of success. In this volume we make the case that manic depression has been a critical factor in propelling some individuals to seek political power, to abuse it, and to become tyrants. Moreover, this book will show that this clinical disorder is the source of many of the irrational characteristics of tyranny.

We shall focus on three men who attained as much power as anyone the world has known—and misused it in so gargantuan a fashion that they became the three greatest killers in history. Napoleon Bonaparte, Adolf Hitler, and Joseph Stalin were champions of death. Napoleon's manic ambitions launched a succession of wars that left millions of soldiers and civilians mutilated, crippled, diseased, or dead in Europe and Russia. Hitler, spurred by manic depression and paranoia, caused the deaths of six million Jews, more than seven million slave laborers, 17 million Germans, and millions more of the soldiers and civilians of the nations that opposed him, including many of the 25 million Russians who died in World War II. Stalin brought about the deaths of more than 40 million of his countrymen through his purges and the famines and other horrors that attended collectivization. What drove them all to power, enabled them to gain it, and then carried them beyond reason was precisely the same disorder—manic depression—which in all three cases manifested itself in startlingly similar ways.

POWER AND DISEASE

As long ago as classical Greece, there was an awareness of sudden mood swings. Manic depression as a medical concept, however, did not emerge until the mid-nineteenth century. In his book *Mood Swings* (1979), the psychiatrist Dr. Ronald Fieve commented that most of society's shakers and doers, whether they be politicians, lawyers, doctors, business people, or entertainers, have some degree of manic depression. In our earlier study, *The Key to Genius: Manic-Depression and the Creative Life* (1988), we explored the contribution that manic depression has made to the lives and works of geniuses in the arts and sciences. Some of the most effective, beneficent, and creative politicians and statesmen in history have also been manic depressives, among them Winston Churchill and Abraham Lincoln. One of the many paradoxes about this illness is that, while it has fueled the careers of many people who have enriched mankind, it has also given genocides to the world.

We shall show how manic depression creates tyrants and the dramatic, unmistakable ways it manifests itself in their day-to-day behavior as well as in their world-shaking, murderous political operations. We shall also describe the essence of the manic depressive tyrannic personality so that people can recognize it. This is especially vital in our perilous era of atomic, chemical, and biological weapons. And manic tyrants seem to gain power in our unsettled, fractious world with alarming frequency. Dictators such as Fidel Castro, Ferdinand Marcos, Muammar Qaddafi, Nikolai Ceaucescu, Saddam Hussein, and many others have been labeled and treated as rational men by journalists and diplomats, yet all have presented many signs of manic depression. After reading the chapters on Napoleon, Hitler, and Stalin the reader should have a greater insight into the aggression, self-righteousness, disdain for others, paranoia, and messianic poses that are the hallmark of the most dangerous forms of the disorder.

Tyrannical manic depressive personalities can also rise to high office in the United States, although American political traditions and the nation's frame of government are more resistant to this. Lyndon Johnson, for example, who had an equally intense lust for power, betrayed many symptoms of mania— egocentricity, incredible energy, volubility, grandiosity—and he, too, developed paranoid convictions.

Why have people of various nations and historical periods submitted to leaders who were manic depressive tyrants? Of course, the people had little choice when they were the subjects of conquest or hereditary monarchs—Ivan the Terrible did not ask for a plebiscite. But time and again, people have endured, even embraced, despots, as the Germans did Hitler. The answer lies partly in the nature of humankind, partly in the nature of manic depression. For one thing, human beings have a strong desire to believe in their leaders. For millennia, people have held a special regard for those who ruled, as though virtue and ability were automatically conferred with power. People want desperately to believe that those in charge are wise and benevolent, protecting them from foreign aggressors and leading them to peace and prosperity. It is intolerable for most human beings to think that the person holding over them the power of life and death may actually be mad.

As a consequence, psychiatric illness among the mighty has been thought to be a rare occurrence. It has been assumed that the psychiatrically ill are too handicapped and too easily identified to ascend to power unless they inherit it. Most people—including many historians—have believed that tyrants are rational men who sometimes make mistakes or are forced into their despotic behavior by historical or political circumstances, or else by some "tragic flaw." This traditional attitude toward despots obscures the fact that the "mistakes" are identical, in many cases, to things that the clinically insane do. There have been two sets of standards for assessing the sanity of rulers and the rest of humankind. Assuming that the mighty have sound reasons for whatever they do, the people have often helped their leaders literally to get away with murder. Those who have dared to say aloud that "the emperor has no clothes" have usually been killed.

Many irrational leaders have been able to fool the world into thinking that they are sane because manic depression is not a conspicuous illness except in its more extreme stages. Manic depressives, for the most part, do not behave in strikingly peculiar ways. The average manic depressive, consequently, is not considered to have a psychiatric disorder. At worst, he may be thought to be moody or hard to get along with. As for people who seek political power, they are generally well aware that their careers would be damaged or destroyed if they were thought to be psychiatrically ill, so they take measures to hide their more bizarre behavior. They withdraw from the public eye when they cannot present a show of normalcy. When they are so ill that they must seek help, they go to medical doctors rather than psychiatrists, and instead of entering a psychiatric hospital, they enter medical hospitals for a socially sanctioned reason such as "nervous exhaustion" or "influenza."

WHAT IS MANIC DEPRESSION?

Manic depression may be defined as a mood disorder with two contrasting states. *Mania* is characterized by expansiveness, elation, hyperexcitability, hyperactivity, reduced sleep, and increased thought and speech. *Depression* is characterized by feelings of sadness, despair, and discouragement, often accompanied by feelings of low self-esteem, withdrawal from interpersonal contact, and such physical symtoms as eating and sleep disturbances and fatigue. In manic depressive disorder, also known as *bipolar disorder,* mania and depression recur in varying degrees of intensity.

Although manic depression is known to be an inherited disorder, the exact mode of genetic transmission has not yet been established. Epidemiologists claim that about one percent of the population will develop this disorder. However, this figure is an underestimate as it reflects only the most severe cases. It does not encompass mild cases that never come to medical attention; moderate cases that are disguised by lifestyle; or severe cases that masquerade as compulsive gambling, substance abuse, or criminal behavior.

Most people are unaware that their thinking and attitudes, their moods, behavior, and personality all depend on the biochemistry of their brains. The biochemistry of manic depression causes abnormal thinking, attitudes, moods, and behavior—it alters the entire personality.

Symptoms of manic depression may emerge in childhood, but it is more common for them to develop, or at least to come to attention, in adolescence or adulthood. Most manic depressive behavior consists of an exaggeration of things that normal people do, especially when they feel intense emotion. Manic depressives are intense much of the time. They may have long episodes of normalcy, and many keep out of view when they don't seem normal, which makes it all the easier for others to be misled into thinking they are merely mercurial. There are many manic depressives who experience only the milder states of mania and depression; therefore, "pass" as healthy individuals.

While manic depressives may not regard themselves as abnormal, they tend to live unstable lives. Their moods, opinions, and even personalities may change rapidly and unpredictably, disrupting friendships and sexual relationships, causing divorce, and estranging them from members of their families. They may not be able to hold jobs and sometimes change their professions. Bankruptcy can be brought on by manic depression because the disorder often interferes with sound financial judgment. All this may happen without the manic depressive's ever realizing what is causing the problems or giving any thought to seeking psychiatric help.

When their disorder enters more severe phases, some manic depressives become prone to physical violence and may spend time in psychiatric hospitals or jails, further disrupting a life already full of uncertainties. People in angry manic states or in agitated depressions are well represented among murderers. Manic depressives are more vulnerable to alcoholism, drug abuse, and compulsive gambling than others; these problems may also afflict members of their families, who often show some degree of manic depression as well. Variable and unpredictable though it may be, however, manic depression is like a lottery—there are prizes for a few.

THE SICKNESS OF THE SUCCESSFUL

While other psychiatric disorders disable or destroy their victims, manic depression sometimes bestows extraordinary gifts on those in its grasp. Mania gives the fortunate ones unlimited ambition and enough confidence in their powers to try to achieve their dreams. It puts the brain into high gear, increasing the speed of the manic's thinking, speech, and everything he does. It floods him with ideas and phenomenal energy. Manic depression cannot substitute for education, innate intelligence, imagination, or talent but it can provide the drive to acquire the first and it can enhance the others. It is the disease of Newton, Beethoven, Mozart, Tchaikovsky, Balzac, Dickens, Goethe, Tolstoy, Kafka, Van Gogh, Monet, and many other creative geniuses.

Manic depression is arguably responsible for the achievements of several of history's great, if often erratic, military leaders and political movers, among them Lord Nelson and Alexander the Great (Goodwin and Jamison [1990]). Manic depression has also produced the great destroyers in history—when in addition to ambition and egotism have been added large measures of ruthlessness, willfulness, utter intolerance of criticism, a consuming need to dominate others, paranoia, and delusions of godlike perfection. Among these we may include the emperor Nero and Mussolini (Goodwin and Jamison [1990]).

The ultimate grandiose delusion that he is an Olympian and that all other human beings are worthless can make the tyrant a champion of death, willing for millions to die if it will further his ambitions. Recently we have witnessed the ascent to power of individuals who are grandiose, paranoid, and despotic, men who have employed threats, brutality, and terrorism to achieve their aims. The loss of life they have caused so far has been limited by their lack of nuclear weapons. But there is no threshold of safety. Even the leader of a small country such as Iraq can constitute a worldwide threat. Humanity will continue to suffer at the hands of the Husseins and the Hitlers, the Napoleons and the Stalins, the grandiose, paranoid tyrants of the present and the future, until this type is so well understood that it can be identified before it menaces the world. This volume was written to promote that understanding.

The final chapter of this book is not only a review of those characteristics of dictators and their governments which are outgrowths of manic depression, but also a manual for the identification of psychotic tyrants. Had Saddam Hussein, for example, been identified ten years ago as a psychotic tyrant, the recent war in the Mideast might have been avoided. Because no one knew what Saddam was, he was given all the help he needed.

Manic depression can strike anyone: it is the bane not only of leaders in politics, the military, and the arts, but also of more ordinary citizens. Their tragedy, however, is equally as great: driven by paranoia or grandiose delusions, they, too, even with their far more limited means, may give vent to their private demons by acts that are antisocial, violent, and even murderous. In a brief epilogue we describe the actions of four figures who have achieved a brutal notoriety in recent years: David Koresh, Jeffrey Dahmer, Jim Jones, and Colin Ferguson. Their crimes are various and many, but, we contend, the underlying cause is the same. A timely diagnosis of manic depression in each could have saved hundreds of lives.

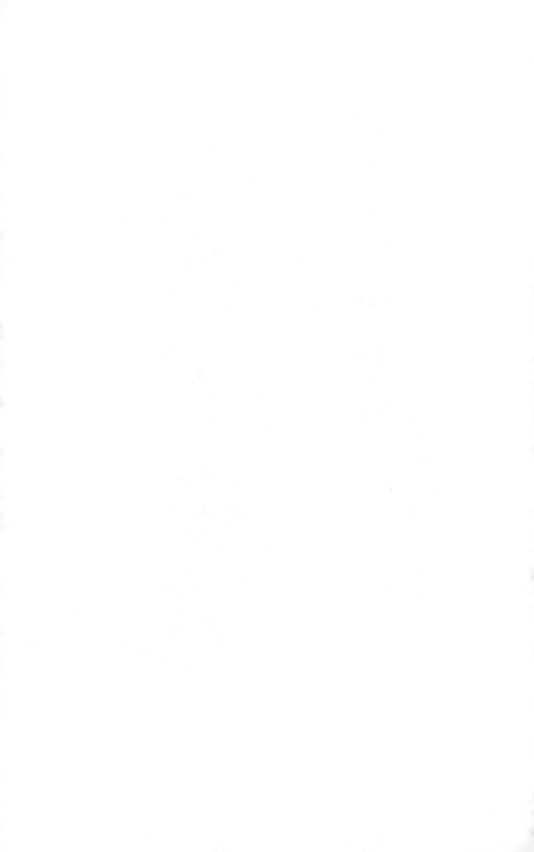

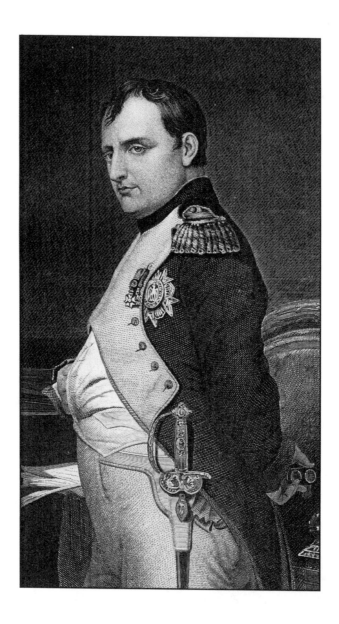

Part One

Napoleon Bonaparte

1

A Self-Made Manic

CHILDHOOD IN CORSICA: 1769–1779

The families of manic depressives are often filled with an assortment of odd and tormented characters who suffer one form or another from the same disease. One brother may be a shrinking violet, an etiolated, gloomy personality wilted by depression; another may be a hothead who expresses his convictions by smashing watches and crockery and anything else in sight. A sister is perhaps a spendthrift with a manic libido, a Messalina who collects and discards lovers as carelessly as ballgowns. The father may be another manic type, a compulsive gambler who lacks the discipline to complete his law degree, leaps into matrimony at an early age, squanders his inheritance entertaining his friends, and, in dazzling displays of impetuosity, fails at everything he undertakes. Such, indeed, was Napoleon's father, Carlo. Such were the sisters and brothers on whom in turn Napoleon would lavish insults, as well as wealth, titles, and kingdoms. Such was the family into which Napoleone Buonaparte, as he was originally named, was born in Ajaccio, Corsica, on August 15, 1769.

Disturbed as his family was, Napoleon proved to be far the most difficult member, the sort nobody would wish on any family. Early on he exhibited the fiery passions of the manic. "I grew up wild and untameable," he wrote years later. Napoleon became wildly infatuated when he was eight years old, trailing his beloved through the streets of the town. He also showed his ferocious temper at an early age. "Nothing overawed me," he wrote. "I wasn't afraid of anybody. I struck one person, I scratched another, 'till all were afraid of me." Greed also surfaced: "I already had the feeling that all that pleases me must be mine." His family called the boy "Rabulione," Corsican for "the one

19

who never minds his own business." Like many manic, driven children, Napoleon slept little, so that neither his mother Letizia nor anybody else got much relief from his frenzied activity.

Letizia Buonaparte and her and her brood suffered most, of course, from Carlo's fecklessness. He commonly spent his evenings and the grocery money at card games when he was not fighting first on one side and then on the other in the inconclusive wars that rent Corsica during the late eighteenth century. Having failed at farming, politics, warfare, and poetry, Napoleon's unstable father died bankrupt.

MILITARY SCHOOLS IN FRANCE: 1779–1785

The Buonapartes spoke a Corsican dialect, and as he was to be educated in a French military school, Napoleon was first sent to school in Autun, France, to improve his French, then to the military school at Brienne, where he stayed for five years. Students and teachers alike found the small, intense young Corsican self-centered, irritable, critical, and morose—all symptoms of depression. A schoolmate recalled him being, "on the whole unpopular with his schoolmates. . . . He had little to do with them and rarely took part in their games." But at Brienne, Napoleon also showed a less disruptive side of his nature, often running off to the library to devour works on history—as he would throughout his life. Far more intelligent and curious about the world than Hitler and Stalin, Napoleon retained a lifelong avidity for books and became one of the better educated men of his day.

Like many manic depressives, the boy easily lost control of himself. Once as punishment for some misbehavior he was forced to eat dinner in the refectory on his knees. He went from rage to vomiting to hysteria, screaming: "I'll eat standing up, Monsier, and not on my knees. In my family we kneel only before God!" When thrown on the floor by the staff and held down he continued to sob, "Isn't that right, Mama? Before God! Before God!"

As Napoleon grew into adolescence, he became even more difficult to like or control, developing a grandiose concept of himself that nothing then or later would dislodge: "From the very beginning I could not bear to be anything less than first in the class," he recalled. In his manic moods, the adolescent Napoleon overestimated his importance to others: "Soon I was the only subject of conversation. I became an object of wonder and envy; I had confidence in my power, and enjoyed my superiority." "Already I had the feeling that my will was stronger than that of others," he continued, and although he knew he was not liked in the school, he consoled himself with the thought that, "I was losing nothing through the indifference of others." In this vaulting sense of Napoleon's own importance and contempt for his fellows lay the seeds of the inhumanity that would later allow him to sacrifice millions of lives for his ambitions.

Napoleon's rebelliousness and ill temper continued during the year that he spent, after leaving Brienne, in military school in Paris. During confession, he argued with the confessor. When rapped on the fingers by a drill instructor, he threw his musket at the man's head. His teachers described him as "capricious, haughty, very egotistical . . . domineering, imperious, and stubborn." By the age of fifteen, the small, dark-eyed youth had developed a personality marked by both manic and depressive traits. Depression made him solitary and silent. Mania made him tyrannical, ferocious, and—most dangerous of all—ambitious.

AS AN ARTILLERY OFFICER IN
FRANCE AND CORSICA: 1785–1793

Depression was for some time dominant in Napoleon's life after his father died of stomach cancer in 1785, leaving the family destitute. Napoleon had his first suicidal urges: "Life has become a burden to me," he wrote, "for I no longer enjoy any pleasure and everything causes me pain." Things did not improve when later that year young Bonaparte left school and joined the army in order to provide some sort of income for his mother, brothers, and sisters. Starting out as a second lieutenant of artillery, he was stationed at Valence, France. For the next seven years, Napoleon traveled frequently between France and Corsica, often returning to his regiment so long overdue that he was once listed as a deserter and was almost cashiered twice. He was too self-willed to make a good soldier and was loyal only to himself. In Corsica he joined the revolutionary forces of Pasquale di Paoli and later fought against them— a turncoat just like his inconstant father.

Napoleon also ended up on the wrong side; in June of 1793, he was forced to flee Corsica with his entire family for exile in France.

During this period of chaos and defeat, Napoleon was plagued by depression. As before, his best friends were books. Devoting much of his small income to his family, he used most of the remainder for reading matter, frequently dining on nothing more than bread and porridge. New clothes were out of the question, so he appeared threadbare as well as hungry. Napoleon spent many of his evenings alone in his room daydreaming about girls or reading. He made no progress with the former, however. Whenever thrown in with people, he bored them with his interminable arguing.

The French Revolution was not his problem: he thought he could not benefit form it, and he was too depressed to enjoy it. The great upheaval that was sweeping France and would, in a few short years, provide Napoleon with his route to power, merely alarmed him at first. He escaped into the study of astronomy during the hours spared from his military duties. "Too many cares spoil my life and influence my disposition," he complained. "They make me solemn beyond my years."

THE CORRIDORS OF OPPORTUNITY: 1793–1796

Solemnity and depression vanished in December 1793, when Napoleon had a chance at the battle of Toulon to demonstrate his soldierly abilities. Commanding the Republican artillery, he was instrumental in driving a British force from the southern French port. Napoleon was one of those for whom the smell of gunpowder and the roar of cannon act like a strong stimulant. Possessed by a furious mania, he showed astonishing courage, along with the energy of a whirlwind, going for days on snatches of sleep while thinking and reacting with lightning speed. His extraordinary performance caught the attention of a man who would be intimately involved with Napoleon's life for some years. The Vicomte de Barras was to become one of the heads of the French government, as well as a lover of Napoleon's first wife, Josephine de Beauharnais. What most impressed the vicomte was the young soldier's "perpetual motion."

The following February, Napoleon was promoted to General of Artillery, but then his career stalled. He had become associated with Robespierre's murderous regime and when it fell, in July 1794, he was jailed for two weeks before being released for lack of evidence. What followed were two years of virtual unemployment, reduced pay, and very dim prospects. Napoleon had made the same fatal mistake as in Corsica: he had backed the wrong side.

As with many manic depressives, misfortune brought thoughts of suicide. He was only "slightly attached to life," he wrote to his brother Joseph. "I shall end by not taking the trouble to get out of the way of a passing carriage."

These dark days were punctuated by violent shifts into mania. Then Napoleon would astonish his acquaintances with, as one witness described it, "moods of fierce hilarity." The manic Napoleon was bursting with strong opinions and harebrained ideas that he flaunted like a peacock's tail. One acquaintance heard him present a "plan of conquest and invasion, which seemed to have been long fermenting in his brain, and came shooting out like lava bursting from the compression of a volcano." At other times, Napoleon longed to go to the Orient, expecting to become commander of the armies of the Turkish Empire.

Napoleon assiduously courted people whom he thought could advance his career, but he was hardly dressed for success. One woman described him as "certainly the thinnest and strangest being I have ever met in my life. The greatcoat he wore was so threadbare, he had such a seedy look, that at first I could hardly believe this man was a general." Another said, "His somber glance made one feel that here was a man one would not care to meet in a forest at night."

Napoleon was too self-centered to notice his effect on people, and this self-absorption was a liability in many social circumstances. He had been trying to make an advantageous match since 1791, but he failed to win the hand of any of his choices, including an aging actress. His fortune-hunting even brought him to the door of an elderly duchess who burst out laughing at his proposal. "But at least think it over," her suitor insisted. She laughed all the more.

However, in October of 1795, an attempt to overthrow the French government opened the door to opportunity in another area. Rebel mobs roamed the streets of Paris. Vicomte de Barras, now a member of the Directoire, France's highest governing body, remembered Napoleon's tireless activity at Toulon and chose him to take care of the rebels. Without a qualm the little Corsican set up his artillery and ruthlessly fired into the approaching crowds. Thus did he gain the government's favor.

In the same year, the young general met his future empress. He was still looking for money or political power or both, and was willing to marry anyone who could rescue him from poverty and anonymity. At last he received an encouraging response from Josephine de Beauharnais, a widow six years older than he, with bad teeth and two children. Her principal attraction was her political influence. She assured him that she could advance his career, and she did. Josephine had been in the beds of Barras, another general, and several other important men. With her contacts, she was able to provide an army for her new lover.

Power, glory, an army! The scrawny young general was driven by joy into mania again and, like many who enter that flamboyant state, succumbed to Cupid. "At last," Napoleon recorded, "things took their course in such a fashion that we fell in love with each other." His manic ardor alarmed Josephine. "Now that I am past my first youth, can I hope that I shall be able to keep alive in him an affection so stormy that it borders on madness?" she wondered. The answer was no, but Napoleon's passion, while it lasted, was intense. "Josephine was at that time a very agreeable lady, full of charm," and also, he added, "had the sweetest little ass in the world." They married on March 8, 1796, and the bridegroom became commander in chief of the army of Italy three days later.

Barras, who had last seen Napoleon in a depressed phase, marveled at the changes that mania wrought:

> Then it was as though he went mad with joy, and whenever he had been dining with me and felt more or less at home . . . he would ask me to have the door closed so that he could give us a play. In this play, which was a genuine improvisation, sometimes on a given theme, he would furnish the dialogue impromptu, taking several parts and acting them all at the same time. He would ask my leave to take off his coat, gather up napkins and tablecloths, make himself different costumes and, after getting behind armchairs to deck himself out, emerge suddenly in the most grotesque disguises . . . he would adopt every tone to vary the different scenes, and with complete success.

Josephine was equally astonished at the heights of mania into which her super-charged Corsican rocketed: "I am alarmed at the energy which animates all his doings."

THE ITALIAN CAMPAIGN: 1796–1797

Napoleon's orders from the Directoire were to drive the armies of the Austrian Empire that were threatening Republican France from positions in northern Italy, but he did not have much to work with. His army was, of all the armies of France, the one in the worst condition: ragged, hungry, and unpaid. Addressing his troops, Napoleon said: "The government owes you much and can give you nothing." But he promised, "I will lead you to the most fertile plains in the world . . . you will find there honor, wealth, and glory." To which an old soldier responded: "His fertile plains are all rubbish. Let him begin by giving us shoes in which to get down to them." Napoleon's generals, seasoned veterans all, were equally unenthusiastic and resented having to obey a 27-year-old neophyte. He convinced them, however, that he would shoot anyone, regardless of rank, who gave him trouble. That settled, Napoleon led his ragged, ill-shod army in one of the most astonishing campaigns of history, utterly defeating the Austrian forces in one battle after another while Europe looked on flabbergasted.

Even these heady triumphs did not keep Napoleon from suffering from the pangs of lovesickness. He was still mad about his wife, who had remained behind in France. "Apart from her I have no gladness," he wrote to his brother Joseph. "She has not merely stolen my heart; she is the only thought of my life!" He kept begging her to join him in Italy and displayed all the wild passion of the manic depressive in love. "Soon I hope to clasp you in my arms, and to cover you with a million kisses as burning as the equator. . . . Heavens! how happy I should be watching you . . . a little shoulder, a little white breast, so firm and so soft."

When Josephine wrote him that she was ill, Napoleon was overcome with anxiety and depression. "My life is one continuous, tormenting dream. A fearful foreboding takes away my breath." To his brother Joseph he lamented: "I am desperate. My wife, all that I love in the world, is ill. I am losing my head. I can no longer stay away from her. If she did not love me, there would be nothing left for me to do on earth." She was, however, perfectly healthy, amusing herself with a lover in Paris. When Josephine finally did join her husband in Italy, in August 1796, she brought her lover with her. But Napoleon was so overjoyed to see her there that he did not notice—at least not at first. By early September, however, he was depressed again, it having penetrated that his wife was not entirely devoted to him. He wrote to the Directoire: "My health is so shattered that I must ask you to find me a successor." By

October, accusing the Directoire of ingratitude and frustrated in his negotiations with Austria, Napoleon threatened to resign: "My health is ruined. I can barely get in the saddle and need two years' rest." So began a pattern common to many manic depressives and recurrent in the life of Napoleon: when anything went awry, depression struck, and he would decide to desert the enterprise which he had begun with much manic enthusiasm.

A TYRANT IN THE MAKING

This first campaign set another pattern for Napoleon. Initially posing as the liberator of the Italian people from Austrian domination, he was hailed as a hero. As he recalled, "the masses surrounded me, shouting 'Evviva il liberator.' " But then his manic greed and ruthlessness earned their hatred. Napoleon made himself (and his family) rich at the Italians' expense while he turned his soldiers loose to plunder city and countryside. In the end he showered the people of Italy with gifts and freedom of a peculiarly Napoleonic variety. He gave them taxes and executions, and freed them from their art works, which went to France. A witness reported: "There was now an end to the shouts and cheers. The farmhand, the workman turned away at the sight of him, and fell back without a word."

Megalomania was also responsible: Napoleon took up residence in a palace. A witness reported: "He was already surrounded by a strict etiquette. His aides-de-camp and officers were no longer admitted to his table. It was an honor much coveted and difficult to obtain. In short, everything had bowed down to the luster of his victories and the haughtiness of his manners."

More important, he ignored the directives he received from the French government, and acted as though he were already King of Italy, a title that he later assumed. Napoleon remarked to an admirer: "Don't you know that there's not one of these directors or ministers but would kiss my boots for 20,000 francs?" To others he confided: "I have never paid the least attention to the plans sent to me by the Directoire. Only fools could take stock in such rubbish." The young general had taken it upon himself to make foreign policy, initiating and concluding wars on his own. It was not enough for him to be the most powerful man in Italy. He was thinking of continents.

"I was only 26," Napoleon later wrote, "but I foresaw what I might become. It was as if I were being lifted up in the air, and the world were disappearing beneath my feet." In addition to this astonishing, monstrous egotism, Napoleon was soon demonstrating the paranoia, grandiosity, and ruthlessness that would mark history's other great tyrants. To attack his reputation, he declared, was to attack that of France itself. In his paranoid moments he saw himself "denounced, persecuted, hounded down by every means." Annoyed by Venice's reluctance to accede to his demands, Napoleon threatened "to obliterate the Venetian name from the earth"—an anticipation of Hitler's and Stalin's policies of group extermination. Napoleon had already begun giving signs of his ambition to rule France, threatening the Directoire with a military coup. "I warn you, I speak in the name of 80,000 men," he wrote. "If you drive them to it, the soldiers of Italy will march . . . with their general; but, if they do, look out for yourselves!"

Napoleon switched to the merry, playful manic when the time for signing peace treaties arrived. One general remembered, "He liked a joke . . . he often joined in our games, and his example on more than one occasion brought the grave Austrian plenipotentiaries to join them also." But Napoleon's moods were, as usual, not to be relied upon; euphoria could suddenly be transformed into rage. At a meeting with the Austrian emissary, Count Cobenzl, prior to the signing of the 1797 treaty of Campo Formio, Napoleon shrieked: "Your empire—it is an old harlot who is used to being violated! You forget that France has conquered and that you are the vanquished . . . You forget that you are conducting conversations with me surrounded by my grenadiers!" Then in his frenzy he smashed an entire coffee service of rare porcelain that Cobenzl had received as a gift from the Empress of Russia. "He behaved," Cobenzl said later, "like a madman."

THE EGYPTIAN CAMPAIGN: 1798–1799

This frenzied anger was succeeded after the treaty was signed by a manic restlessness and boredom. In peace there was no action, no fame. "All things fade here, and my reputation is almost forgotten," Napoleon wrote, also complaining that "I no longer have any glory: this little continent of Europe doesn't provide me with enough of it. I must go to the Orient: all the great glory comes from there."

The result was Napoleon's strange, misbegotten invasion of Egypt. The idea in part, like Hitler's adventures in Africa 140 years later, was to strike at the British Empire, a risky undertaking at best. The French had a large fleet in the Mediterranean, but it was no match for the Royal Navy. Some members of the Directoire approved it largely because they now feared the upstart Napoleon and hoped he would deposit his bones in Egypt.

Napoleon, on the other hand, driven by a manic optimism, saw the invasion as "the means by which I could carry out all that I had dreamed." He went into a fever of planning and preparation. No one else was permitted to exercise any authority. His orders were so detailed that they even specified how many socks each soldier should bring along. The general and his army sailed from Toulon on May 19, 1798. They stopped at Malta where, during a six-day whirl of manic energy, Napoleon set records for benevolent interference. He abolished servitude and freed 2,000 slaves, established fifteen primary schools, ended feudalism, and gave Jews equal rights with Christians. Landing in Egypt, Napoleon continued his manic activity. He presented himself as a liberator of the people from their feudal lords, the Bey-Mamelukes. In quick succession he established a postal service and a mint, erected street lamps in Cairo, founded a hospital for indigents, began a stagecoach line between Cairo and Alexandria, and boasted that he would build the largest mosque in the world. To pay for this, Napoleon extorted huge sums from the Egyptians, and pillaged whole towns and villages. To discourage an uprising, he held executions, cutting off heads, he boasted, "at the rate of five or six a day."

Depression intervened briefly when Napoleon at last learned about his wife's infidelity. "The veil has been torn assunder," he wrote his brother Joseph. "You are the only person remaining to me: I treasure your friendship. . . . Arrange for me to have a country house when I return, either near Paris or in Burgundy. . . . I am weary of human nature. I need to be alone and isolated. . . . Great deeds leave me cold. . . . Fame is insipid." Fame soon recovered its seductive charm, but Napoleon never again allowed a woman to take advantage of him.

His marriage, however, was the least of his problems. The English had caught him in a trap of his own making. Napoleon realized that his campaign was doomed when the British fleet, having defeated the French at the Battle of the Nile, began to patrol the Egyptian shore, making it impossible for his forces to receive supplies or reinforcements from France. However, his mania returned and he decided to leave the Near East by way of Syria. This was not a solution to the shortage of supplies, but he still fancied himself another Alexander the Great and intended, like Alexander, to invade India. Napoleon also expected to dispose of the Ottoman Empire on the way. His was a grandiose, wildly impossible strategy, as the French soon found out. The decisive battle took place at the Syrian city of Acre. Even while losing it, Napoleon boasted to his old friend and private secretary, Louis de Bourrienne: "I will cause all Syria to revolt and provide it with arms. I will found in the Orient a great, new empire that will fix my place in posterity; and perhaps I shall return to Paris via Adrianople or Vienna, after having destroyed the House of Austria." It was another manic dream. The sum of his accomplishments in the sands of the Levant was the execution of 4,000 prisoners of war who had been promised their lives, and the slaughter of the inhabitants of the city of Jaffa.

NAPOLEON'S FIRST DESERTION OF HIS TROOPS

Two days later Napoleon's mania had subsided, leaving him rational enough to order a retreat. The trek across the desert back to Cairo was a plague-ridden nightmare. More than half the army, some 20,000 men, died. Napoleon, in a suicidal mood, needlessly handled the flea-infested, abscessed corpse of a soldier stricken with bubonic plague. Unfortunately, the Black Death refused his invitation. Instead, relief came in the form of news that French forces were being defeated in Italy; furthermore, the political situation in France was in flux. This provided Napoleon with an excuse to desert what was left of his army in Egypt. He would return to recapture Italy. He concluded, with his habitual humility, that it was also time for him to take over the government in Paris. The Corsican justified his decision to rule France by saying: "Large battalions are always in the right."

Bonaparte sneaked away without even saying goodbye to General Jean-Baptiste Kleber, whom he left in charge of a hopeless cause. Kleber became enraged when told Napoleon had left, and said: "The man has gone off like a second lieutenant who leaves unceremoniously after having filled the cafes of the garrison with the noise of his humming and his debts." This was not only an accurate assessment of the way Napoleon departed from Egypt, but also a good simile for the way Bonaparte would lose other wars. Some months afterward, the critical Kleber was assassinated and the remnant of the army surrendered.

Long before then, Napoleon had sailed for France, arriving on October 9, 1799. Although he had destroyed an army and deserted the remnants, he was still a hero to the French public. He himself believed the disaster was no fault of his own, and learned nothing from it.

NULLIFYING THE FRENCH REVOLUTION

Napoleon was almost undone by his own ungovernable emotions when he overthrew the government of France by a *coup d'état*. He had wanted the legislature to elect him to rule over them. When the members refused, Napoleon lost control, screaming: "Caesar, Cromwell, tyrant—that is all I have to say to you! Liberty! Equality! You forget the Constitution! Hypocrites! Intriguers! I will abdicate power the instant the Republic is free from danger. The gods of fortune and war are with me!" Urged by one of his supporters to calm down, Napoleon only got worse, shouting at his generals: "Follow me. If they resist, kill, kill! I am the god of the day!" The situation was saved when his brother Lucien, who was president of the Assembly, called in some of Napoleon's troops. In an atmosphere of chaos and gunpowder, the five members of the Directoire and France's two legislative bodies, the Council of Elders and the Council of Five Hundred, were forced to resign and General Bonaparte was elected one of three consuls to rule the country. The other two consuls were merely "consultative."

A subsequent general election established a new constitution that empowered Napoleon to appoint people to every position of importance in the government, the military, and the Church. The date was December 24, 1799, and France was his. The century had ended, the Revolution with it, and gone were the liberties for which so many had sacrificed their lives.

The First Consul's will became law. Within months Napoleon had shut down all but four out of France's 73 newspapers. On being told that some members of his new government objected to his establishment of special courts, he replied, "What should stop me from having them all flung into the Seine?" When his brother Lucien asked if he was not "afraid that France may rebel against your shameful abuse of power," Napoleon chillingly replied, "Never fear, I shall bleed her so white that she'll be incapable of it for a long time to come."

The bleeding began almost immediately. The new First Consul proposed peace to France's inveterate enemies, England and Austria. Both refused. It had not escaped their notice that on the same day he issued the peace proposal Napoleon had told his army, "Soldiers! It is no longer the frontiers of the Republic which you are called upon to defend. We must invade the territories of our enemies!" The result was a new series of battles that—at the cost of many French lives—again sent the Austrians reeling back through northern Italy. More fighting gained Napoleon parts of Holland, Belgium, and Germany.

At home another sort of bloodletting followed a bomb attempt on Napoleon's life. The botched assassination plot gave him the opportunity to purge one wing of his opposition, the Jacobins, who hated him for revoking the freedoms and civil rights won by the Revolution. Napoleon did away with numbers of the Jacobins without the nuisance of holding trials. A short time later, the actual terrorists confessed that they had acted on behalf of royalists who wanted to restore a Bourbon king to the throne. Without showing a trace of regret for having executed the wrong men, the First Consul bellowed that he would have vengeance on the Bourbons, too.

Tyrannical at home, Napoleon for a time played the statesman abroad. During this period he made some of his most brilliant political moves. First he signed peace treaties with all the former enemies of France except England. After that, he astutely made peace with the pope through a concordat that restored the privileges of the Roman Catholic Church in France. Although Napoleon was not sufficiently magnanimous to restore church property confiscated during the Revolution, the agreement gave him the support of the clergy and of millions of French who had remained devout. The following year, Napoleon even made peace with England. He also arranged to have himself elected sole consul, to hold the office for life. There was no power left in France that could curb his will.

IN THE MOOD FOR WAR: 1803

Success, however, is as dangerous to a manic depressive as failure. The latter can bring on overwhelming depression; success can ignite mania, and that can lead to delusions of omnipotence. "Europe," a manic Napoleon said, "is an old, rotten whore. I have 800,000 men. I shall do what I please with her." This he undertook to do, initiating what turned out to be thirteen years of almost continual war, during which he built and destroyed an empire.

His temper completely out of control, Napoleon began in a thoroughly manic way, ranting at a British envoy, Lord Whitworth. During a first meeting, on February 18, 1803, he screamed at Whitworth for two solid hours in the presence of the terrified diplomatic corps. "Do you want war?" he yelled. "We have been fighting for fifteen years. That's far too much. But you want fifteen more years of war and you are forcing me into it!" Then Napoleon turned to the Spanish and French ambassadors, saying, "The English want war, but if they are the first to draw the sword, I shall be the last to sheathe it!" A second encounter took place a month later. In front of 200 guests at the Palace of the Tuileries, Napoleon again raged at Whitworth about English perfidy, then walked out. A third meeting was less stormy but did nothing to erase the ambassador's memories. Reporting to England, Whitworth concluded, "I am persuaded that the First consul is determined to avoid a rupture if possible; but he is so completely governed by his temper that there is no possibility of answering for him." Britain's leaders correctly deduced that they never could conclude a lasting peace with Napoleon, although they did not yet fully realize the extent of his irrationality.

After he annulled the treaty of peace he had made with England, Napoleon told the French that he had chosen war "only with the greatest repugnance." But to confidants he revealed his deepest desire: "In three days' time, given some foggy weather, I can become the master of London, Parliament, and the Bank."

He soon did something that made him an object of loathing across the entire Continent. Reacting with fury to the news of several plots to kill him, Napoleon ordered the arrest and execution of a supposed conspirator, the Duc d'Enghien. This was unwise for three reasons. First, the duc was a popular member of the nobility. Second, it became clear that d'Enghien was innocent. Third, Napoleon had him seized and murdered outside of French territory by secret agents. Napoleon shrugged off the incident, saying, "Pooh! What is one man after all?"

What he never realized, with his contempt for human life, was the effect that this crime had on his fellow Europeans. With this one act it became clear that Napoleon's whims were lethal, and that no man, woman, or child living anywhere was safe from his thugs. "The murder of a young prince beloved by all Europe," a contemporary noted, "excited universal disgust."

2

"Where the Possible Left Off"

Not content with being consul for life, Napoleon wanted to make his office hereditary, like that of Europe's other monarchs. To that end, on May 18, 1804, he proclaimed himself emperor. He could have settled for "king," but manics are rarely troubled by modest ambitions. Following the example of Charlemagne, he had to be crowned by a pope, so he summoned the pontiff to Paris for an elaborate coronation ceremony. At the climactic moment, as the pope was about to place the crown on his head, Napoleon suddenly took it and crowned himself. This classical example of manic egotism and impulsiveness inspired a popular poem:

> On loans and aims I long supported life,
> I fawned on Barras, took his whore to wife,
> I strangled Pichegru, shot Enghien down,
> And for so many crimes received a crown.

The day after the self-coronation, the new emperor was no longer satisfied with being merely an emperor. He complained that nineteenth-century Frenchmen were unlikely to worship him as a god: "I came too late. . . . Yes, I admit that I have had a fine career, I have gone far. But what a difference with antiquity! Look at Alexander: when he had conquered Asia and presented himself to the nations as the son of Jupiter, the whole Orient believed him. . . . Well, if I announced that, every fishwife would hoot when she saw me pass by. The masses are too enlightened these days; nothing great can be done anymore."

31

Not that his subjects' englightenment earned his respect. The distended ego of the manic leaves no room for such sentiments. Napoleon thought of his fellow citizens as pernicious children without sense or any rights—"an assemblage of undisciplined men," he said, "who soon become undisciplinable if they are not restrained by a hand of iron."

While Napoleon scorned the people of his nation, he insisted they render him homage. French children were taught to say: "We owe him love, respect, obedience, fidelity, military service, and all the tributes ordered for the defense of the empire and throne, and fervent prayers for his welfare." And what the French did today, the world would do tomorrow. A courtier reported, "Napoleon entertained the strongest conviction of his being destined to conquer every nation of the globe."

THE BEGINNINGS OF SELF-DESTRUCTION: 1805

The self-destructiveness inherent in such blinding ambition, however, was already beginning—even in this summer of his power—to eat away at Napoleon and his regime. For one thing, his bellicosity—his manic, driving will—would not allow him to remain at peace with the rest of Europe. Soon France was at war again with a powerful coalition of Prussia, Russia, and Austria while the hostilities with England continued unabated. And while Napoleon won a great many victories, including the triumph of Austerlitz, each battle cost France and its armies men and materiel that would mount, in time, to unaffordable losses.

On the home front Napoleon weakened his regime from within by choosing flagrantly incompetent aides and advisors. Manic depressive dictators habitually surround themselves with people of that caliber in preference to those who are capable and qualified. The manic's ego dooms his own regime. His paranoid suspicions, need for constant praise, and his jealousy of anyone possessing real ability, ensure that the capable will soon depart and the second-rate will stay. One of his ministers observed that once Napoleon was emperor, he "hit on the idea of molding a generation of satellites. He often said that men of forty were imbued with the principles of the old regime, and therefore could not be devoted to his own person or principles. He took a dislike to them, and from that moment started a nursery of 500 or 600 young men, whom he appointed in turn to every office. . . . Not all these young men had either the capacity, or the prestige, or the decorum required. But he thought them devoted to his person and government, and that was enough." Only yes men and sycophants were permitted to remain for very long in Napoleon's inner circle. The minister added, "All about him were timid and passive. They studied the will of the oracle and performed it blindly." Hitler and Stalin would surpass even Napoleon in their recruitment of the execrable.

By 1805, Napoleon's megalomania had determined his fate: the monarchs of Europe would combine to eliminate him. He made it evident that they must fight or be conquered. When he thought Austria was arming he declared, "I want her to disarm; if she won't, I shall pay her a little visit with 200,000 men which she will not soon forget." From that moment, no state in Europe could increase its forces without finding itself at war with the Corsican and if it failed to arm, it would end under his heel anyway. He also made it clear he intended to dethrone Europe's ruling houses. Dispensing entirely with discretion, Napoleon boasted to the Austrian Prince Metternich, sent as an envoy by his enemies: "Before another ten years mine will be the most ancient dynasty of Europe." It did not require much subtlety to realize that Bonaparte intended to unseat and possibly kill all the Continent's remaining royalty.

A FATEFUL FOLLY: 1806

In 1806 Napoleon conceived another grandiose project, a continental blockade. No English ships would be permitted to land anywhere on the coasts of Europe, nor English goods permitted entry. Moreover, all Englishmen on European soil were to be arrested and their possessions confiscated. Since he did not actually control all of Europe, it was impossible for Napoleon to enforce his blockade. Eventually he had to violate it himself in order to procure supplies for his armies. Despite the failure of the blockade to bring England to her knees, it was sufficiently effective to ruin trade and cause financial hardship throughout Europe, increasing hatred for the man who imposed it.

Napoleon was an exceptionally intelligent man and a moment's dispassionate consideration would have convinced him that the blockade was an egregious folly. But he was acting under the delusion that he could accomplish anything he wanted. He also entertained another manic delusion—that he was innocent of all wrongdoing, which he attributed to others. "It is the English," he insisted, "who have compelled me to expand constantly. If they keep it up, they will oblige me to annex Holland!"

This in fact he did, making his brother Louis king of the Dutch. He also gave his brother Joseph the kingdom of Naples. Napoleon selected them for kingship not because of any respect for their native ability. He believed they would simply be more compliant than people who were not relatives. They surprised him, however, by taking their responsibilities seriously and trying to look after the welfare of their subjects. This outraged the emperor. "Remember," Napoleon admonished Louis, "that you are first of all, above all, a French prince. I placed you on the throne of Holland merely to serve the interests of France, and to second me in all I am doing for her." Brother Louis replied: "To be sure, my heart is still French, but the day I have to sacrifice Holland to your schemes, my rule will be over."

On hearing this, Napoleon, his fury mounting, berated his brothers and sisters for their lack of gratitude. A witness described the imperial fireworks: "Amid the dazzle of a thousand candles, the blaze of diamonds and other jewelry, men in uniform were drawn up in rows, between which Napoleon was striding up and down. His features were swollen and almost deformed with rage. . . . His brother Louis was trying to keep up with him." The court of a manic depressive does not lack for entertainment.

DEBACLE IN SPAIN, THE POPE IN PRISON: 1807–1809

By 1807, Napoleon had as much power and territory as he could win and more than he could control. He ruled directly—or through his puppets—France, Belgium, much of Germany, Italy, Austria, Poland, all of Holland, and Switzerland. He might have held on to what he had won if he had convinced the monarchs of Europe that his ambition was finally satisfied. But he never made the effort. Instead, his megalomania drove him to invade Portugal on the pretext that the Portuguese were violating the continental blockade.

In 1808 Napoleon also seized the Spanish throne by treachery and threats of royal executions. Then he placed his good-natured but reluctant brother Joseph upon it. Bonaparte gave the same justification for his Spanish adventure as he had for his invasion of Portugal: violation of the continental blockade. It seems never to have occurred to him that the blockade was costing too much and proving unenforceable. Mania sustained Napoleon's faith in his omnipotence. He announced, "God has given me both the inclination and the power to surmount all obstacles."

With all these aggressive moves, Napoleon carelessly squandered the lives of soldiers whom he would sorely need later on to defend his own throne. The Spanish adventure was a constant drain as guerrilla bands relentlessly fought the French occupying forces. "This miserable war has ruined me," Napoleon complained. "It has complicated my troubles, divided my forces, and destroyed French morale in Europe." On learning that Spanish guerrillas were defeating his best troops he flew into a rage and smashed crockery. But it never occurred to him to bring his soldiers home. Though others bled, his grandiosity remained unscathed. When Napoleon was told that the Chinese worshiped their sovereigns as gods, he responded, "That is as it ought to be."

In 1809, Napoleon erased perhaps his finest stroke of statesmanship, the concordat. Five years earlier, he had told French officials to treat the pope with the respect due to a man who had the moral equivalent of 200,000 troops to back him up. This was a realistic assessment of the power of the Catholic Church. But Napoleon was no longer dealing with reality. Deep in manic delusions of godlike power, he no longer cared how many enemies he made.

Seizing the territories in Italy ruled by the pope, he deposed the pontiff and made him prisoner. Bonaparte's public explanation for this folly was that the pope did not respect the continental blockade. His real reason, unbelievably, was that he wanted to take the pope's place. "Paris would have become the capital of Christendom," he recalled on St. Helena, "and I would have become master of the religious as well as the political world. I would have called religious as well as legislative bodies into session; my church councils would have been representative of all of Christendom, and the popes would have been mere chairmen." Only a madman would think that he could imprison the pope and then be accepted by Roman Catholics throughout the world as Christ's Vicar.

INVITING BETRAYAL

Napoleon was isolating himself from men who had hitherto been his most loyal and effective counselors and aides. One of France's best generals, as he was dying, found the courage to say: "Your ambition is insatiable, and it will be the end of you. Unsparingly and unnecessarily, you sacrifice the men who served you best; and when they did, you feel no sense of loss." The general's analysis was correct. Napoleon's manic ego decreed that all others were merely disposable and replaceable instruments of his will.

He finally made the error of alienating his invaluable foreign minister Talleyrand. Working himself into a rage, Napoleon screamed at his minister, "What are your schemes? . . . I should break you into a thousand pieces, and I have the power to do it. But I despise you too much to take the trouble. Do you know what you are? You're a turd in a silk stocking!" For three hours, Napoleon continued this intolerable abuse of a man who had helped him rise to power. Subsequently, in the manic delusion that outrageous treatment had no effect on people's loyalty to him, Napoleon sent Talleyrand as his emissary to Tsar Alexander. Talleyrand begged the tsar to save Europe from the insanity of the French emperor, and later joined openly with Napoleon's enemies.

The emperor concluded this year of manic self-sabotage by divorcing Josephine. In retaliation, she told people that her husband was little better than a eunuch. Six days after the divorce she wrote him: "Public consideration, which you urge as the ground for deserting me, is a mere pretense on your part; your mistaken ambition has ever been, and will continue to be, the guide of all your actions—a guide which has led you to conquests and the assumption of a crown, and is now driving you on to disasters, and to the brink of a precipice."

THE NEPHEW OF MARIE ANTOINETTE: 1810–1812

The year 1810 was another one of mania, in which Bonaparte was living on just three or four hours' sleep a night. He was excited by his newest project: a second and much more illustrious marriage. He wanted instant nobility and found a wife who would make him both a Bourbon and a Hapsburg, the nephew of Louis XVI and Marie Antoinette. His prospective bride, Marie Louise, was the daughter of Austria's Emperor Francis I. She was not enthusiastic about the match. For as long as she could remember, her suitor had been her father's worst enemy. However, her father could not afford to refuse a man who defeated him so regularly, and the marriage was arranged.

The bride was young and not unattractive, and for a while the emperor was once again the passionate lover that manics often become. A lady of the court recorded: "For the first three months after his marriage Napoleon was at the empress's side day and night. The most urgent business could hardly tear him away for a few moments. . . . All were surprised at this alteration. The ministers were uttering cries of protest. Old courtiers watched and said that this state of things was too violent to last."

While it did last, Napoleon was a charming husband. Marie Louise, who had expected the worst, was swept away by his euphoria and wrote home:

> When I left you and my friends at Vienna, I saw the good people plunged in the deepest sorrow, from a persuasion that I was going to a sacrifice to my new destination. I now feel it an agreeble duty to assure you that during three months' residence at this court, I have been and am the happiest woman in the world. From the first moment I met and saw the Emperor Napoleon, my beloved husband, he has shown me, on every occasion, such respectful attention, with every token of kindness and sincere friendship, that I should be unjust and ungrateful, not to acknowledge his noble behavior.

Notwithstanding the delights of this amorous interval, the newlywed husband had blind rages in which he so panicked some spectators, including generals, that they became paralyzed by fright and had to be helped out of sight before the emperor thought to order their arrest. One witness wrote: "I still ask myself what was Napoleon's nature, that he could pass so abruptly from the intoxication of love to that of wrath and fury. It was the nature of the volcano: Etna roars while covered with flowers."

Eventually, the roses of romance wilted and the young empress discovered what kind of man she had married. Napoleon's feelings also altered. He said later, "Frequently, I would have liked to divorce her."

In 1811, Napoleon and Marie Louise toured Belgium. There was a striking difference in people's attitudes toward husband and wife. She was received, an onlooker recorded,

> with great applause. The emperor got very little. It had been heaped on him in 1803. But the captivity of the pope, the threat to religion, the devastation of Spain and the odious abduction of its king, the total coercion of the press, the repeated conscriptions, the warrants, the banishments, and the kidnappings of children had made a remarkable change. People were gasping under that huge pressing machine known as the French Empire. . . .

Bonaparte, regardless, had the manic delusion of being loved. Sinking deeper into fantasy, he announced, "In two years time I shall possess the entire world." The arrival of a son made the father yet more grandiose. "I envy him!" Napoleon said of the infant. "Glory awaits him, but I had to pursue it. I was Philip, he will be Alexander. He has only to reach out his arms to seize the world." Napoleon insisted that his courtiers bow to the cradle and read speeches to the infant. Even Napoleon's sycophants found his behavior excessive. "The emperor is mad—completely mad," one of them wrote. "He will throw all of us, such as we are, head over heels, and the whole thing will end in a catastrophe."

It was a timely prediction. Napoleon's mania was about to accomplish what none of his enemies had been able to do alone or in combination— exterminate his army. The seed of his undoing was his conviction that conquering Russia would help him defeat England—a mistake repeated by Adolf Hitler. Napoleon's ostensible justification for the invasion was the usual one: Russia was violating the continental blockade. Mania made him blind to the risks involved, but no one dared to point them out. He had instructed his ministers that they should not aspire to independent opinions, for even to doubt him was equivalent to betrayal.

According to his valet, Constant, this was a period of fierce elation for Napoleon. "He never whistled so much, and was never so gay, as just before he set out for the Russian campaign." Napoleon was also foolhardy. Heretofore a master planner of campaigns, this time he did not even ensure a secure base of operations or a safe supply line. He decided that the conquest of Russia would make him "Emperor of the West," so he ordered coronation robes to be packed in his luggage. But he did not bother to order winter clothing for his troops. He had not a single doubt that he would conquer Russia before the cold winds of autumn blew.

3

"From the Sublime to the Ridiculous"

THE ROAD TO MOSCOW: 1812

The first days of the march to Russia presaged what was to follow. Napoleon fell off his horse. Extremely superstitious, the emperor regarded this trivial incident as an evil omen, and depression replaced the manic confidence that had spurred him to undertake the invasion. As the Grand Army crossed the Polish border, Napoleon remained morose and silent, unable to make up his mind whether to move on into Russia or winter where he was. Having decided to proceed, he saw his troops decimated by disease as much as by combat. By the time the Grand Army arrived at Smolensk, 120,000 men had already been lost.

At Borodino, as usual, the prospect of battle made Napoleon manic. He greeted the dawn with "Here is the sun of Austerlitz!" expecting to repeat that great victory. But by midday he became sullen, inert, indecisive, and despairing. Disabled by depression, Napoleon shirked his responsibilities as commander, refusing to answer questions or give orders. Ultimately, he abandoned the battlefield. "One could see him either seated, or slowly walking back and forth," a witness remembered. "When almost at every moment messengers brought him news of the loss of his generals, he only made gestures of sad resignation." "I do not recognize him," one of his generals said. Bonaparte still might have won a decisive victory by sending his Imperial Guard into action, but his depression kept him from issuing the order, despite the urgings of his generals, until it was too late to make a difference. Borodino was at best a Pyrrhic victory for the French. The carnage on both sides was shocking and Napoleon lost forty of his general officers.

38

MADNESS IN MOSCOW

Once the Grand Army had struggled on to the Russian capital, Napoleon's condition became even worse. Moscow was in truth depressing enough. Most of its citizens had fled and the Grand Army entered a ghost town. Napoleon spent his first night there in the sleeplessness of anxiety. Mysterious fires broke out all over the city. Again, Napoleon was seeing omens: "This forebodes great misfortune for us," he said. Depression deepened his pessimism, and the expectation of failure deepened his depression, trapping him in a vicious, downward spiral. An assassination attempt by a Russian youth intensified Napoleon's feeling of hopelessness. "His eyes, usually so bright, appeared dim and languid," recorded General Armand de Caulaincourt, "and an indescribable expression of uneasiness was depicted on his countenance."

Napoleon sank into a devastating, incapacitating depression that brought a multitude of symptoms, both mental and physical. Though gifted with a marvelous memory he had periods when he forgot important dates and names, even confusing one person with another. He suffered from stomachaches and malaise. "The emperor seemed overcome with fatigue," his valet Constant noted. "From time to time he clasped his hands over his crossed knees, and I heard him each time repeat with a kind of convulsive movement, 'Moscow! Moscow!'" Stuporous, silent, Napoleon stuffed himself with food. He became unkempt, withdrawn, incapable of work or discharging essential responsibilities, and indifferent to what was happening around him. A severe depression can make life difficult under the best of circumstances. Here was an army commander, deep in enemy territory, responsible for the survival of half a million men, disintegrating before the horrified eyes of his generals, with no one permitted to take his place.

Without warning, this paralyzing depression would flash briefly into mania. Napoleon's wild instability made reasoned decision impossible; when he was not prey to the hopelessness of depression, he was absurdly optimistic. What remained of his thinking now was steeped in fantasy. He sent emissaries to the tsar with offers of peace under the manic delusion that he and Alexander could still be friends. Rebuffed, he made impossible plans to revenge himself on the tsar by capturing St. Petersburg. Napoleon also went to concerts, lingered over meals, read novels, discussed the finer points of poems, or the doings at the Comédie Française—anything to avoid confronting the terrible reality of extricating his army from its desperate situation. Unable to accept losing so little as a chess game, Napoleon could not accept that the conquest of Russia was beyond the reach of his still formidable army.

When he did rouse himself to give orders, they were absurdly impractical. He instructed his supply officers to purchase 20,000 horses and enough provisions for two months although he had already been told that his foragers were unable to find so much as one day's rations in a countryside long since stripped of everything useful by the enemy. Napoleon knew all this because he had seen how barren the country was as he passed through it. Ordering horses and supplies was more than wishful thinking; it was a delusional denial of desperate conditions.

In the end, Napoleon's delusions and shifting moods prevented him from making the decision that would have saved what was left of his forces. He could have left Moscow in early October and brought his men out of Russia before the rigors of winter caught them. Instead, he did nothing. In all, thirty-nine days went by during which Napoleon was too mentally ill to lead his army.

DEATH MARCH

When the depression lifted and freed Bonaparte from his lethargy, he ordered retreat to begin on October 19. As Hitler's generals were also to discover, winter arrives in northern Russia with ferocious finality in early November. And the army did not begin its long march through ice and snow alone. Napoleon's forces were harried by marauding Cossacks and constantly had to fight minor engagements with the Russian horsemen. But the deadliest enemy was winter, blanketing everything with snow, killing men and horses with cold, disease, and starvation. Arctic temperatures forced the weakened, exhausted men to abandon weapons and supplies, and drove many to escape their suffering by committing suicide. By the time the Grand Army had reached Smolensk, half of the hundred thousand men who left Moscow were already dead or missing.

Then on November 6, in the midst of the horrors of the retreat, Napoleon received a dispatch from France that, Constant noted, made him "very merry." There had been an attempted *coup d'état* in Paris. Like the news of troubles that had come to him during the Egyptian retreat, this offered him an exit from the despair and death all around him. He could leave the disasters behind and return to Paris on the excuse he was needed there.

By the end of the month he was planning to abandon his miserable, dying troops. "Cold and privation have broken up the army," he said. "Possibly the army cannot be rallied short of the Nieman. In this state of things, I may decide that my presence in Paris is necessary for the safety of France, of the empire, of the army itself." Napoleon then sent a bulletin to Paris that gave an all too clear picture of the destruction of the Grand Army. It was not, of course, his fault. The disaster, he wrote, was entirely due to the early arrival of winter. Nothing he said later suggests that he ever regretted the loss of his army or the suffering and demise of over half a million men. The last words of the bulletin were gems of egotism: "Never has His Majesty been in better health." That should make up for everything.

Napoleon deserted his men under cover of darkness after bribing his staff with hundreds of thousands of gold francs. "By daybreak the army had learned the news," Constant recorded, "and the impression it made cannot be depicted. Discouragement was at its height; and many soldiers cursed the emperor and reproached him for abandoning them." The army he left behind degenerated into a demoralized mob, the survivors fighting each other over what little food and shelter they could find.

Bonaparte reached Warsaw on December 10, where his minister to the King of Saxony, Abbé de Pradt, observed and recorded the emperor's psychotic conversation. The two men met at the hotel in which Napoleon had paused for refreshment. When they were joined by two members of the Polish government, Napoleon asked, "How long have I been in Warsaw? Eight days —No, only two hours . . . from the sublime to the ridiculous there is but a step." "Dangers! Not the least," Napoleon continued. "Agitation is life to me: the more trouble I have the better I am. None but sluggish kings fatten in their palaces. Horseback and camps for me. . . . I am more wanted on the throne than with my army. I leave it with regret. All that has happened is nothing; it is misfortune; the effect of climate. The enemy is good for nothing: I beat him everywhere." Napoleon cheerfully added, "It was written in heaven that I should marry an archduchess." He also exclaimed several times, "I was told every morning that I had lost 10,000 horses during the night— Well! bon voyage." After rambling on for another three hours, Napoleon concluded: "I never was better; if I carried the devil with me, I should be all the better for that."

Napoleon remained manic all the way to Paris. General Caulaincourt, who accompanied him, had to endure a jocular, endless, and, at times, grotesque harangue. On entering Prussia, the emperor said, "Can you picture to yourself, Caulaincourt, the figure you would cut in an iron cage, in the main square of London?" Caulaincourt responded, with what might have been double entendre, "If it meant sharing your fate, Sire, I should not complain." "It's not a question of complaining," Napoleon went on, "but of something that may happen at any moment." He added that Caulaincourt would be "shut up like a wretched Negro left to be eaten by flies after being smeared by honey." This sadistic fancy kept Napoleon laughing hysterically for the next quarter of an hour. When they arrived at the border of France, Caulaincourt thought the emperor more lighthearted than he had ever seen him before. A bereaved nation was waiting.

ONWARD TO ELBA: 1812–1813

Back in his capital, Napoleon was still in the grip of mania. The day following his arrival, he worked for fifteen hours, sending out a stream of orders and letters. Constant, who reached Paris a week after his master, recalled, "The emperor was very gay and seemed to have forgotten all his fatigues. I said to him that everywhere my eyes had been struck by the same frightful spectacle. . . . I had seen the dead and the dying, and poor unfortunates struggling hopelessly against cold and hunger." Napoleon told Constant to "go rest, my poor boy."

Even more astonishing, Napoleon, the master strategist, had learned nothing from the greatest military debacle the world had ever seen. Although it had just been proven beyond any rational doubt that Russia was invincible, its vastness swallowing up any invading army sooner or later, Bonaparte insisted, "If the Russians had not burned Moscow I would have been master of Russia." His manic ego would not permit him to believe anything else. Of the Grand Army, only about 4,000 men remained. No horses were left, hence Napoleon had no cavalry. Nevertheless, he threw himself into plans for his next war. Before long, his savagely efficient police had rounded up a new army of nearly half a million soldiers, many of whom were adolescents barely out of childhood. He would lead them marching off to the same fate that had consumed their fathers and brothers.

Faced with a conquest-mad Bonaparte, a new alliance of European states declared war on France in 1813. The spring of that year saw Napoleon fighting both the Prussians and the Russians. A meeting called to discuss peace terms—France desperately needed an interval between wars—found Napoleon in a raging mania. The allies, he screamed at Metternich, would need "to mobilize millions of people and shed the blood of several generations" in order to conquer Napoleon. "I grew up on a battlefield," he said, "and a man like me cares little for the lives of a million men." "Do you think," he continued, "you can overthrow me by coalition? Well, how many allies are you? Four, five, six, twenty? The more numerous you are, the less I shall worry." He later explained, "The fact is I never intended peace at Prague."

Napoleon might have survived had depression not intervened again. Fighting against several allied armies in Germany, he was immobilized at Dresden for a month. Once more as in Moscow, a stupefying depression paralyzed his mind. He slept excessively, passed his waking hours reading, and ignored messages. He was incapable of giving orders. He could not make up his mind what to do or where to march the army next.

Depression crushed him again at Duben two months later. He became totally incapacitated and spent two days in a mental fog. Caulaincourt recorded:

> His eyes were dim and fixed. . . . His hands were convulsively agitated, and he took up and threw down unconsciously any object that happened to lie within his reach. . . . I approached him and said, "Sire, this state of mind will kill you." He made no reply. . . . All my efforts to rouse him were

unavailing. His faculties seemed suspended. . . . throughout the following day the emperor's mind was racked by anguish and indecision.

This kind of depression, for which the technical term is "retarded," turns the brain into something like a factory in which all the power has been cut off and the workers either sit idle by their machines or grope their way slowly through dark rooms. The manic afflicted with a retarded depression becomes almost unrecognizable.

"His character seemed utterly changed," noted an astonished Constant. "Who would believe it? To the activity which drove him on, and so to speak, incessantly devoured him had succeeded a seeming indifference which is perfectly indescribable. I saw him lie on a sofa a whole day, the table before him covered with maps and papers at which he did not even glance, and no other occupation for hours than slowly tracing large letters on a sheet of white paper."

THE EMPIRE CRUMBLES: 1813–1814

Napoleon refused to consider making peace even after the French suffered a severe defeat at the hands of Swedes, Austrians, Prussians, and Russians at Leipzig, on October 19. His generals recognized that he had passed far beyond the bounds of reason and was leading them to destruction. One of them said to another the next day: "Couldn't you see, in these last events and the catastrophe that followed, that he'd lost his head? The coward, he was deserting us, sacrificing us all."

The emperor had, indeed, deserted his army for the third time, again running off to Paris. There Napoleon, although the tide of war had clearly turned against him, entered another period of intense mania. Even Constant, who had seen it all, was amazed at this new frenzy of activity that, he said, "far from diminishing, seemed to increase each day." Telling the Senate, "Nothing on my part is hindering the re-establishment of peace," Napoleon was demanding the conscription of 110,000 more recruits and the levy of new taxes to pay for this army. After a member of the Senate commented, "For the last two years, we've been harvesting men three times a year," Napoleon dissolved that body.

By early spring of the next year, Napoleon again in the grip of battle mania, with only 47,000 of his own men, took on an Allied army of 230,000. His generals had abandoned all hope, but the magic of mania made Napoleon feel and even look young again. Constant said, "The emperor, in proportion as the danger became more pressing, displayed still more his energy." And as long as he remained manic, Napoleon kept winning. He became so optimistic that he talked about invading Russia again. But though the emperor was his old self, albeit temporarily, France had changed. The young and the strong were dead. His generals were begging for "peace at any price." Disregarding them, a manic and grandiose Napoleon refused to end the war unless he could dictate all the terms. The very mania that gave him such advantages in battle doomed him to waste his victories and destroy his empire.

ABDICATION AND POISON

Eventually, however, the mania passed and the victories stopped. By March the Allies were advancing on Paris. Napoleon, restored to sobriety, at last realized that he might win many battles and still lose the war. Briefly he considered letting the Bourbons resume the throne. Constant noted, "His Majesty was extremely agitated, and spoke in such broken tones that I understood only those words which he repeated many times: "Recall them myself—recall the Bourbons! What would the enemy say? No, no! It is impossible! Never!"

Napoleon retired to Fontainebleau. When the Allied forces reached Paris, he concocted a plan to drive them away. But the fire had gone out of him. His wife, son, and brother had fled Paris, a provisional government was in place, and his generals refused to continue the war. Constant recorded, "the emperor became each day more sad and careworn. . . . From time to time I heard stifled sighs . . . often he did not notice the arrival of persons whom he had summoned, looked at them, so to speak, without seeing them, and sometimes remained nearly half an hour without addressing them; then, as if awakening from this state of stupefaction, asked them questions without seeming to hear the reply. . . ." One day Napoleon "had torn his leg with his nails until the blood flowed, without being aware of it," the valet noted.

By April 13, the emperor had abdicated, taken poison, taken an antidote, and was manic again. He went around the palace whistling a dance tune. With groundless optimism, he expected his wife and son to join him there.

The mania was replaced by a state of extraordinary instability. The following description of Napoleon's behavior, recorded by his valet, would in itself justify a diagnosis of manic depression. Only manic depressives undergo such extreme and abrupt shifts of mood without external cause. Constant noted:

> He appeared calmer and more cheerful than for a long time past. . . . However, this gaiety was only momentary; and, indeed, the manner in which the emperor's mood varied from one moment to another during the whole of our stay at Fontainebleau was perfectly indescribable. I have seen him on the same day plunged for several hours into the most terrible depression; then, a moment later, walking with great strides up and down his room, whistling or humming . . .; after which he suddenly fell into a kind of a stupor, seeing nothing around him, and forgetting all the orders he had given.

When Napoleon received letters from Paris, Constant adds, "his agitation became extreme—I might say convulsive."

Napoleon would never see his wife or son again. Defeated and taken prisoner, he headed for exile on the island of Elba on April 20, 1813.

4

The Naked Emperor

THE EMPIRE OF ELBA

It is an irony of history that the man designated by his mother to be the savior of Corsica, and who had tried to become ruler of the world, was made by the clemency of his enemies the sovereign of Elba, a tiny island off the southern coast of France. While being escorted to his new realm, Napoleon became lighthearted and joked, "After all, I've lost nothing. For I began the game with a six-franc piece in my pocket, and I've come out of it very rich."

This mood soon changed. As Napoleon was passing through France on his way to exile, he encountered hostile Frenchmen who hanged him in effigy, yelled curses, and tried to attack his carriage. He cowered out of sight, behind one of his generals. Depressed again, he made himself a disguise and, when the party stopped at an inn, refused to eat for fear of poison. He had weeping spells that lasted for hours.

Once he was safe on shipboard, the pendulum of his moods swung once more. Entering another interval of mania, Napoleon became quite cheerful, looked healthy, laughed at witticisms about his past, and deluged the ship's English captain with nautical questions. Upon landing on Elba, he gaily challenged the captain to a gallop around his diminutive kingdom.

Bonaparte was usually manic in any novel place or situation, at least until the novelty wore off. His high mood persisted during his first months on the island. He surrounded himself with mistresses who doubled as ladies-in-waiting. His mother and sister Pauline also kept him company. He had a complete court in miniature, including a grand marshal of the palace. He even had a tiny navy and a little army which he reviewed often.

His mania kept Bonaparte from feeling any embarrassment at his fallen state. He gave fêtes of all kinds and held audience with tourists. Rising before dawn, he rushed about all day and gave balls at night. He started the construction of roads and fortifications. An English colonel noted: "I have never seen a man in any situation of life with so much personal activity. . . . He appears to take . . . much pleasure in perpetual movement, and in seeing those who accompany him sink under fatigue." The colonel added ominously, "His thoughts seem to dwell perpetually on the operations of war."

With the obdurate optimism of the manic, Napoleon clung to the expectation that his wife and child would return to him. By September 20, he had abandoned that hope and a lethargic depression had returned. A witness noted, "He occasionally falls into a state of inactivity . . . and has of late retired to his bedroom during several hours of the day." Bonaparte made these sad days as short as possible and went to bed early.

But relief was coming, in the form of news that the emperor's replacement, King Louis XVIII, was increasingly unpopular. If Napoleon wanted to return, now, it appeared, was the time to do it. He was not a man to waste an opportunity to seize power. His spirits rose again, he planned his escape, and decamped from Elba on February 26, 1815. By good fortune he avoided the British navy while crossing the Mediterranean, and landed on French soil quietly, with a handful of followers, on March 1. History was giving Napoleon a second chance. But manic depression did not.

ENCORE: MARCH–JUNE 1815

As Bonaparte made his way toward Paris, soldiers and civilians eagerly attached themselves to his cortege. The emperor, in the time-honored tradition of politicians seeking supporters, made all kinds of promises he did not intend to keep. He declared that he would reduce taxes, restore freedom, and adopt a liberal constitution. Even the forces sent to capture him joined him. Napoleon later confessed that any resistance at all would have stopped him, but there was none.

Louis XVIII sped out of the country before Bonaparte reached Paris. Without firing a single shot, Napoleon overthrew the King of France and on March 20 was carried back to power on the shoulders of cheering crowds. None of his victories had inspired such enthusiasm in the people of France as did his return from defeat and exile. They made a tragic mistake.

The emperor was manic again, in "rapture," a witness said, "being gay to a degree of madness." Napoleon got up at one or two o'clock in the morning to work and was busy all day. There were moments of euphoria, as when visiting an orphanage full of admiring children he said, "This is the acme of bliss—these are the happiest moments of my life." He shed tears of joy when he left the orphan girls who had cut off pieces of his coat for souvenirs.

But mania brought back the same mad ambitions and grandiose delusions. "I wanted the kingdom of the world," Napoleon said. "The world summoned me to rule it. . . . If I had remained on the throne I would have died with the reputation of being the greatest man that ever lived."

On the first day of his second reign, Napoleon had declared, "No more war, no more conquests. I mean to reign in peace, and to make my subjects happy." But the day after his return to Paris, he began assembling another army. When a delegate from the Institute of Sciences said some time later, "the nation is looking forward to peace," the war-loving emperor turned purple, shouted "Peace!," and gave the man a kick.

Napoleon was aware that the people of France did not want a return to tyranny and tried to create the impression that the days of dictatorship were over. "I busied myself with the constitution on my return from Elba just to be in fashion," he later admitted. He permitted only inconsequential changes to be made in the edicts governing the empire. "From that moment," recalled a member of the government, "Napoleon was seen as an incurable despot. For my part, I regarded him as a madman bound hand and foot and delivered up to the mercy of Europe." Talleyrand also regarded Napoleon as a maniac and refused an offer of millions to rejoin the government.

Once the novelty of his return to power wore off, however, Napoleon's mania departed and his depression returned. Weariness, hesitation, and apathy overwhelmed him again; he often slept fifteen hours at a stretch. While mania had lifted him to the apex of power, manic delusions lured him to destruction. Depression was about to render the *coup de grâce*.

On June 14, 1815, the emperor and his newly formed army crossed the Belgian frontier to meet the British and Prussian armies sent to oppose him. Four days later he lost the battle of Waterloo, although he had more men and more artillery than the opposing forces. He was defeated not only by the British Duke of Wellington, but also by the disabling depression that had seized him before the battle. At one point Napoleon refused to issue orders and became disoriented. At another, he wanted to lead a suicidal charge against the enemy. Once more Napoleon refused to face the consequences of defeat. Deserting his battered troops, he raced back to Paris in three days and sleepless nights.

Shocked to see him in the capital, his supporters urged him, "Don't stay an hour! Go at once! Go to the head of your army!" Instead of heeding their advice, Napoleon explained that several other people were to blame for Waterloo, then took a bath. As always, on escaping from a defeat with a whole skin, Napoleon enjoyed an interval of mania and when manic he saw the world as he desired it to be. He had been informed months earlier that the English were planning to confine him on the island of St. Helena if they caught him. He had also been warned that the Prussians would shoot him if they go him first. Nevertheless, his manic imagination convinced him that he would be allowed to keep his throne as long as he did not leave town. Later on he admitted, "A schooboy would have been brighter than I."

Beguiled by his incredible conviction, he relaxed for a week, talked about going to America, and received farewell visits from former mistresses. He entertained visions of himself as a humble cottager in England and invented a pseudonym for that role: Colonel Mueron. However, Napoleon did one practical thing: he misappropriated three million francs in gold that belonged to the treasury of France. By June 23, Napoleon had realized that his enemies would not permit him to remain emperor. He abdicated for the second time, in favor of his son, Napoleon II. But even this was too optimistic; no Bonaparte was acceptable as ruler of France. This second abdication had the same denouement as the first: the return of Louis XVIII to the throne.

Finally acceding to the pleas of his supporters, Bonaparte left Paris on June 29 and headed for the coastal port of Rochefort. The escape from Paris achieved nothing because for three days he was unable to decide what to do next. It no longer mattered. Napoleon had allowed so much time to go by that the English now controlled the entire coast of France. Escape was no longer possible. Under the manic delusion that reality would conform to his plans, Napoleon wrote a letter to the British Prince Regent demanding asylum in England. Then he confidently delivered himself over to a captain of the British navy.

THE PRISONER: 1815–1821

Aboard the English ship *Bellerophon* as a captive, Napoleon, seemingly oblivious of the circumstances, was in good humor, and charmed the ship's officers. At meals he asked "many questions," the British captain said, "about the manners, customs, and laws of the English; often repeating . . . that he must gain all the information possible on those subjects, . . . as he should probably end his life among that people." Napoleon was slow to abandon this fantasy. When informed officially that the British were shipping him to St. Helena, he raged, denying he was a prisoner and demanding that he be accorded the rights of a British citizen. "I will not go to St. Helena," he swore over and over. "I prefer to redden the *Bellerophon* with my blood."

But go to St. Helena he did, and there repeated the pattern he had displayed on Elba: a massive denial of reality. In his new captivity he insisted on the same formalities as when he ruled Europe. Members of his party had elaborate titles. There was a "Grand Master of the Palace," although no palace existed. One person served as Finance Minister, Minister of the Interior, and Minister of External Affairs because of the shortage of personnel in Napoleon's entourage. Fortunately, this shortage was matched by the shortage of things for them to do. There was no longer an empire to administer. Dependent though he was on his small band of followers for companionship and various services, Bonaparte disregarded their feelings and dominated them mercilessly, even exacting sexual favors from the wife of a member of his retinue. She bore Napoleon a daughter.

His companions in exile found Napoleon's moods and behavior as unpredictable and inexplicable as ever. On good days he would go around singing old operatic arias. Receiving newspapers, one of his few contacts with the outside world, could set off a brief manic episode. A companion observed: "At these moments he was not the same man as before; his bearing, his voice, his gestures, all showed that fire was circulating in his veins; his imagination became excited to such a point that he became a supernatural man. He seemed still to command Europe." Dictating, like other kinds of work, could still make Napoleon temporarily manic. One day he dictated for fourteen hours at a stretch and felt no fatigue when he was done. He also became manic over new undertakings, no matter how trivial. When he took up gardening he would spring out of bed before sunrise and rouse everyone else as well. Whatever project was in train, Bonaparte would do the planning and issue orders while others did the work.

The exile's paranoia was nourished by his confinement. Although the British maintained Napoleon with great generosity, spending millions of pounds on him and his retinue, he complained constantly that he was receiving less than his due. He also accused the British of seeking his blood, claiming that they had chosen St. Helena as his place of exile so that its climate could kill him. The climate had no observable effect on either Bonaparte or any member of his court-in-exile. Subdued at last by cancer, he died on May 5, 1821.

The tyrant's corpse returned in triumph to France on December 15, 1840. The cheering crowds had short memories, but a member of his government knew what kind of hero this was: "The outcome of all his wars, and of what he called his glory, has been to deprive us of conquests rightfully made before his name was heard . . . and deliver us up to two invasions by all the nations of Europe."

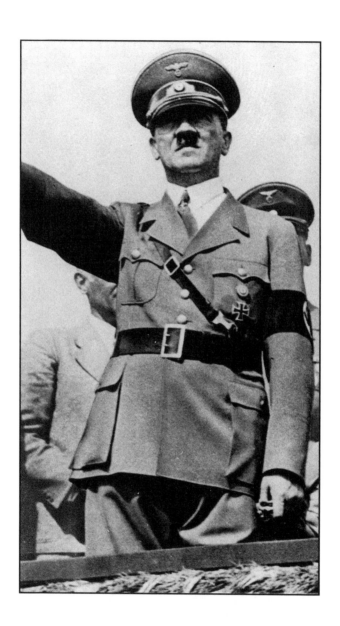

AP/Wide World Photos

Part Two

Adolf Hitler

5

The Changeling

THE DEFORMATIVE YEARS

Adolf Hitler was born on April 20, 1889, in Braunau, Austria-Hungary. Like Napoleon's, his was a troubled, unstable family. His alcoholic father, Alois, married three times, twice to women already pregnant by him. He had mistresses as well, illegitimate children, and was himself the son of an unwed mother. He was 52 when Adolf was born. He died thirteen years later.

The father and his two sons, Adolf and his half brother, Alois, shared a number of the defects common to manic personalities, including the impulsiveness and restlessness that are so disrupting to family life. The father continually changed residences, sometimes twice in one year. The older brother, Alois, became a drifter and spent periods in jail for bigamy and theft. All three men shared another manic affliction: ungovernable anger. Hitler recalled, "I never loved my father. . . . He had a terrible temper and often whipped me." Alois left home permanently at age fourteen because of conflicts with their father.

Life in this ferocious family was not easy for Hitler's mother, Klara, a passive farm girl considerably younger than her husband. She favored her son Adolf over her daughter and two stepchildren although he was difficult as a young child, his character already distorted by some of the manic depressive traits he was to exhibit throughout his life. "He was imperious and quick to anger from childhood on and would not listen to anybody," his half brother, Alois, recalled. "He would get the craziest notions and get away with it. If he didn't have his way, he got very angry. He would fly into a rage over any triviality. He had no friends, took to no one, and could be very heartless." The egotism and arrogance of the tyrannic personality were already in evidence.

The manic's irresistible urge to talk appeared in Adolf's penchant for lecturing trees and making speeches on empty hilltops at night. He was also an aggressive child. His favorite pastimes were war games, which he continued to play after the other boys his age had outgrown them.

A good student until he reached the age of eleven, the boy then added another manic trait to his repertoire and became rebellious. One of his teachers described him as:

> certainly gifted, although only for particular subjects, but he lacked self-control, and to say the least, he was considered argumentative, self-opinionated, willful, arrogant, and bad-tempered. He had obvious difficulty in fitting in at school. . . . He demanded of his fellow pupils their unqualified subservience, fancying himself in the role of leader. . . . He reacted with ill-concealed hostility whenever a teacher gave him some advice.

The resentment of other people's knowledge or authority never left Hitler, who remained throughout his life unwilling to learn from anyone else. Consequently he never developed; he merely aged.

Although he had periods of manic busyness, schoolwork did not excite the young Hitler and he was not a diligent student. Too unstable to discipline himself, he could only work when in the mood. By the time he was sixteen, he wanted no more of school. "One can learn much better by oneself," he told his mother. Whatever she may have thought, the widow put no obstacles in the way of her domineering son and allowed him to quit.

The previous year, while living in Linz with his sister and mother, Hitler had met the one really intimate firend he ever had—August Kubizek, an upholsterer's son. The boys were close in age and both were passionately devoted to music. August studied piano, but his family expected him to join his father's trade, for which he was being trained. Hitler was supposed to become a baker. The desire to choose their own courses in life was another bond between the two adolescents. During the four years the boys were together, Hitler revealed himself completely to his friend. A memoir Kubizek wrote years later provides the earliest, clearest picture of Hitler's mind and behavior.

Kubizek, who was both sensible and perceptive, quickly realized that there were two Hitlers. One was remarkable for his "ecstatic dedication and activity," Kubizek observed, while the other had "dangerous fits of depression" so severe that they isolated Hitler from all human contact for weeks at a time. Kubizek often saw him "sit alone on his bench in the Schonbrunn Park, holding imaginary conversations with himself." When depressed, Hitler "was inaccessible, uncommunicative, and distant," Kubizek attested. "Adolf would wander around aimlessly and alone for days and nights in the fields and forests surrounding the town. . . ." If Kubizek asked him what was wrong, Hitler replied, "I don't know myself."

Hitler sometimes found temporary relief from depression in music, particularly that of Wagner, which could even lift him into a manic mood in which he concocted grandiose political plans and subjected his long-suffering friend to interminable declamations. "I soon came to understand that our friendship endured largely for the reason that I was a patient listener," Kubizek observed. "I remember how he used to give me long lectures about things that did not interest me at all. He just had to talk." Kubizek recognized the compulsive element in the manic's pressure of speech. "These speeches seemed like a volcano erupting," Kubizek continued. "Such rapture I had only witnessed so far in the theater, when an actor had to express some violent emotions. . . ."

Kubizek also witnessed the explosive irritability which occurred during Hitler's periods of mania and depression. "Adolf was exceedingly violent and high-strung. Quite trivial things, such as a few thoughtless words, could produce in him outbursts of temper . . . quite out of proportion to the significance of the matter. . . . There was no end to the things that could upset him."

The teenage Adolf did nothing to support his mother, whose only income consisted of the pension she received as a widow; nor did he look for a job or seek training of any sort. He was already so estranged from reality that he could not fit himself into the workaday, practical world—and he never did so. But he enthusiastically threw himself into unlikely projects when the frantic, driven, ceaseless activity of mania seized him. It was, said Kubizek, "as though a demon had taken possession of him. Oblivious of his surroundings, he never tired, he never slept."

Grandiosity was another early sign of Hitler's manic depression. He spent months making drawings in which he redesigned the buildings of the town of Linz. Although he had no training in architecture, he never doubted that his adolescent plans and designs would be executed. Hitler kept his drawings, and when Austria became part of the Third Reich thirty years later, Linz was reconstructed according to the ideas he had set down at the age of sixteen. History must have a sense of humor.

Hitler believed in his own omnipotence and was convinced that for him nothing was impossible. "He did not know what resignation meant," Kubizek recalled. "He who resigned, he thought, lost his right to live." This is one of the manic delusions that can sustain tyrants during setbacks in their struggles for power.

The manic's egotism and need to dominate were also evident in the adolescent Hitler. Like Napoleon, he wanted exclusive and complete possession in a relationship. Kubizek remembered that his "claims on me were boundless and took up all my spare time. . . . I had to be at his beck and call. . . ." Hitler told him: "I can't bear that you should mix with other young people and talk to them."

THE DILETTANTE

Hitler's lifelong infatuation with art began in adolescence. He would, he told Kubizek, devote his life to writing poetry, to drawing, to painting, to going to the theater and attending the opera. Hitler's creative production never amounted to much, but even when he was Chancellor of Germany he fancied himself as primarily an artist.

When he was sixteen, he took his first step toward a career in the arts— he refused to begin an apprenticeship to a baker. His mother capitulated to his insistence that he must go to Vienna to attend art school. Unwilling to go alone, Hitler succeeded in persuading the Kubizeks to send August to study music in Vienna. In this instance, August was grateful for Hitler's interference: a career in music was what he wanted most, and he attained it.

Living in a large, cosmopolitan city changed Hitler not at all. As before, he threw himself into all sorts of odd projects that mania convinced him he could accomplish. In addition to redesigning the architecture of Vienna, he attempted to invent a substitute for alcoholic beverages, then devoted his time to a substitute for tobacco. He drew up a program of school reforms and worked on designing a new kind of government for Germany. Kubizek noted: "Although he had learned nothing and achieved nothing, he rejected all advice and hated instruction. Knowing nothing of composition, he took up an idea Richard Wagner had dropped, and began writing an opera . . . occasionally, too, he painted. . . . Incessantly he talked, planned, raved, possessed by the urge to prove he had genius."

THE MAD ROMANCE

At seventeen Hitler fell in love for the first time. The romance became a wild journey into delusion. Undeterred by the fact that his beloved Stefanie never spoke to him or took notice of him, he wrote her a flood of love poems and fervently believed that they communicated telepathically. "Adolf was always sure that Stefanie not only knew his ideas exactly," Kubizek recalled, "but that she shared them enthusiastically. . . . He expected Stefanie to reciprocate his love for her to the exclusion of all others. . . ." She went out with young officers only so that she could disguise her true feelings, Hitler thought. None of this was expressed to Stefanie, who became engaged to someone else.

The engagement threw Hitler into a suicidal frenzy. "I can't stand it any longer!" he screamed. "I will make an end of it!" This was the first of many suicidal declarations. "He was unable to work or even think clearly; he feared he would go mad," Kubizek noted. Hitler drew up elaborate plans for himself and Stefanie to jump from a bridge into the Danube.

Another adolescent excursion into fantasy revolved around the lottery.

Filled with manic certitude that he would win, Hitler bought a ticket and, Kubizek remembered, "was at once transported into a future where he occupied the third floor of a house on the bank of the Danube. He spent weeks deciding on the decor, choosing furniture and fabrics, making sketches, and unfolding . . . his plans for a life of leisure and art." When Hitler failed to win, "he flew into a rage. Significantly, it was not only his bad luck at which he stormed," Kubizek noted; "he denounced human credulity, the state lottery organization, and finally condemned the cheating government itself." Like other psychotic manics, Hitler believed that whatever he desired would come to be and reacted to disappointment by encasing his ego in an armor of paranoia and rage.

DEFEATED BY REALITY

It had been Hitler's intention to enroll as a student in the Vienna Academy of Arts, but he failed the entrance examination. A second blow fell three months later: after four years of widowhood, Hitler's mother died on December 21, 1907, of cancer of the breast. Hitler was seventeen.

He did not abandon his goal, however. In February of the next year he took some private art lessons to prepare for the Academy examination which he planned to take again the following September. Kubizek, who had benefited from a good musical education before he came to Vienna, was already matriculated in the Vienna Academy of Music. Unlike his grandiose friend, Kubizek was progressing so well that he had his own music students.

In moments of manic optimism, Hitler declared that the coming revolution would eliminate the necessity for a diploma and his lack of training would not stand in the way of a career as an architect. When depressed, he complained "that bad luck was pursuing him; that there was a great conspiracy against him—he had no possibility of earning any money." Although the conspiracy was a figment of paranoia, Hitler's architectural drawings display a talent that might have been adequate for a career in art had he had suitable instruction. His failure to gain entry into art school was not his tragedy alone.

During this period in Vienna Hitler developed a fervid interest in politics. He and Kubizek attended a performance of Wagner's *Rienzi,* and Hitler left the theater in a manic excitement. "Now he aspired to something higher," Kubizek wrote. "He was talking of a *mandate* which, one day, he would receive from the people, to lead them out of servitude to heights of freedom." In 1939, Kubizek visited Hitler for the first time since their days together in Vienna. The dictator told his boyhood friend: "In that hour it began."

When a second attempt at the Academy examination resulted in lower marks than the first one, Hitler fell into a severe paranoid depression. "He wallowed deeper and deeper in self-criticism," Kubizek recalled. "Yet it needed only the slightest touch . . . for his self-accusation to become an accusation against the times, against the whole world; choking with his catalogue of hates, he would pour his fury over everything, against mankind in general who did not understand him, who did not appreciate him, and by whom he was persecuted. I see him before me, striding up and down . . . in boundless anger."

Hitler's anti-Semitism was part of this hatred and paranoia. By the time they were in Vienna, Kubizek remembered, Hitler's bigotry, noticeable before, had become a raging obsession. Unable to admit to himself that his talent or training might be insufficient, he blamed the Jewish members of the Academy faculty for keeping him out of art school. He wrote to the director of the Academy, "For this the Jews will pay." In later years he told people, "I really wanted to be an architect. The Vienna Jews knew how to stop that."

If Kubizek had been refused admittance to the Academy of Music, perhaps he and Hitler would have stayed together longer. As it was, Kubizek's success was more than Hitler could endure. In November 1908, Hitler vanished from Kubizek's life without a word of warning and could not be found. Though he was still in Vienna, Hitler had entered another world, that of the hopeless, the hungry, and the penniless. It was *The Beggars' Opera* come to life.

"VERY CLOSE TO MADNESS"

After fleeing from his successful friend, Hitler led a completely solitary life in a succession of rented rooms until his small inheritance was exhausted. In the autumn of 1909, he went to a charity ward and sank into a dreary hand-to-mouth existence, picking up odd jobs, begging money for food, or eating at soup kitchens. None of this was caused by his economic circumstances; Hitler was eligible to draw an orphan's pension sufficient to maintain him in modest comfort, but he neglected to collect it. His depression was so severe that he was unable to take care of himself or to meet even the simplest demands of ordinary life. He somehow lost or abandoned almost all his possessions, including his overcoat. He became filthy, his hair grew to his shoulders, a beard covered his face, and his clothing turned to rags. During these months he experienced a fathomless misery that he would always remember with horror.

By 1910, the depression had diminished somewhat and Hitler was able to move to better quarters. There he was able to earn some money painting cheap posters and post cards that a fellow vagrant named Hamish hawked for a commission. Hamish complained, though, that Hitler "was never an ardent worker, was unable to get up in the morning, had difficulty getting started, and seemed to be suffering from paralysis of the will." These symptoms of depression were relieved on occasion by manic days during which the silent Hitler became a domineering fanatic who ranted about politics and went into frenzies. Then, instead of filling orders for post cards, he concocted schemes for becoming wealthy overnight. His manias, however, did not last long enough for him to attempt to build any of his castles in the air.

By the spring of the following year, Hitler had emerged from his depression to the point where he dressed in passable clothing and became more disciplined in his work. During his more manic moments he elaborated his political philosophy. In 1912 he decided that all German-speaking peoples—Austrians, Swiss, Transalpine Italians, with assorted Czechs and Poles—must be welded into a single German nation, which would then dominate Europe.

That same year, without a word of explanation to anyone, he went to England, where he stayed with his half brother, Alois. On arriving, Hitler was noticeably depressed, apathetic, unkempt, and sank into the lassitude of a stuporous depression again. He spent most of each day on a sofa, made no acquaintances, and learned no English. He later improved enough to leave the house, which he did primarily to take walks alone. After four or five months Hitler returned to Vienna and resumed painting post cards. His sometime agent Hamish, seeing him oscillate between lethargic depression and manic agitation, considered him "very close to madness."

His own paranoia and bigotry finally drove Hitler from Vienna. He had come to hate the city for what he called its "mongrel" population. Moreover, he never forgave Vienna for witnessing his humiliation and disintegration. When the war brought bombing raids to Vienna, Hitler punished the entire city by refusing to give it adequate anti-aircraft protection. In May 1913, he went to Munich, thinking he would be happier in a truly German city. But he felt no better there. Depression imprisoned him in his room for days at a time and he spoke to no one.

A STRANGE HERO

What saved Adolf Hitler from this dreary, aimless life was World War I. It gave him a purpose. Victory for Germany was more than just his private fantasy; he shared it with an entire nation. Moreover, war gave him a community to belong to: the German army.

But even in the army Hitler continued to be something of a pariah. His exaggerated, unpredictable moods set him apart and he made no friends. A fellow soldier recalled that "he sat in a corner, with his helmet on his head, buried deep in thought, and none of us was able to rouse him from his listlessness. . . ." Another remembered Hitler spending "hours by himself, his head down, never speaking a word." The future führer refused to join other soldiers for conversation or any social activity.

When he was not totally withdrawn, he was overactive, intrusive, making speeches or having sudden rages. "We all cursed him and found him intolerable," a member of his company later said. Nevertheless, Hitler performed well in battle and received commendations for bravery. He later spoke of his war years as being overwhelmingly happy.

During the war Hitler experienced hallucinations that bulked large in his later thinking. "I was eating my dinner in a trench with several comrades," he later wrote. "Suddenly a voice seemed to be saying to me, 'Get up and go over there!' It was so clear and so insistent that I obeyed automatically. . . . I rose at once to my feet and walked 20 yards along the trench. . . . Then I sat down to go on eating. . . . Hardly had I done so when a flash and deafening report came from the part of the trench I had just left. A stray shell had burst over the group in which I had been sitting, and every member of it was killed." This well-timed auditory hallucination contributed to Hitler's grandiose belief that he would survive every danger, every threat to his life, until he had fulfilled what he conceived his mission to be.

During the last months of the war Hitler experienced another influential hallucination. He was lying in a hospital recovering from a leg wound, exposure to mustard gas, and a temporary blindness attributed by his doctors to hysteria. Severely depressed, he was thinking about commiting suicide. Hitler recovered his vision in the hospital, but when news came that Germany, already losing the war, was being wracked by rebellions, he was overcome by a fit of weeping and a second attack of blindness followed by the hearing of voices calling him to save Germany; Hitler also found his blindness leaving him. "Suddenly," he said, "the idea came to me that I would liberate Germany, that I would make it great. I knew immediately that it would be realized." This conviction hardened his earlier dreams of being Germany's Joan of Arc into the resolution to enter politics instead of devoting his life to architecture. This decision, made in a psychotic state, would bathe the world in blood.

6

"A Master of Irrationality"

CREATING THE NAZI PARTY

The war over, Hitler found employment as a spy for what remained of the German army, gathering information about groups that the army considered subversive. One of these was a small, militant circle of malcontents who, like many other Germans, blamed the loss of the war on "traitors" and Jews. Finding kindred souls, Hitler stopped spying, joined the group, and was soon elected as one of its speakers, his specialty being his anti-Semitic harangues. Occasionally his manic fury was an impediment. "He got into such a rage," a witness said, "that people at the back couldn't understand very much."

Despite this handicap, Hitler soon became an important figure in the movement—with the help of its leader, Dietrich Eckhardt. Eckhardt took the former post card painter in hand, tutoring him in proper dress and manners. He also introduced Hitler to some rather high social circles, to the people who would help finance the new National Socialist, or Nazi, party. By 1921, Hitler felt strong enough to demand he be named party president, and he was.

The astonishing growth of the Nazi party in the early 1920s was due in part to Hitler's gifts as a mesmerizing orator and his talents for publicity and political organization. Contributing as well was the Nazis' willingness to use violence to suppress rival groups. Hitler proclaimed in January 1921: "The National Socialist Movement in Munich will in future ruthlessly prevent— if necessary by force—all meetings or lectures that are likely to distract the minds of our fellow countrymen." That September, he and two other Nazis attacked a man who was giving a speech, beating him with sticks and chairs until he fell from the platform. Hitler declared: "It's quite all right. We did what we had to do." He spent a month in jail for the assault.

A necessary condition for the movement's success was the matching of the man and his times. Except for medals won during the war, Hitler's life had been a series of defeats. Now he lived in a country that was defeated, too. The poisonous resentment and bitterness that his own life had brought him could now be shared with and expressed for the German people. This was no minor political asset. Even Hitler's often bizarre behavior failed to disillusion the faithful who flocked to the swastika banner that the führer himself had designed.

As the Nazis gained power and wealth, Hitler's life became more gratifying than it had ever been before. But these improvements still failed to alter his character or diminish his paranoid hatreds. Through the 1920s and into the 1930s, Hitler was little changed from the orphaned and rejected adolescent August Kubizek had known. Manic depression still ruled. "He is such a nice man," one of his landladies remarked, "but he has the most extraordinary moods. Sometimes weeks go by when he seems to be sulking and does not say a word to us. . . ." An English reporter who interviewed Hitler in 1923 found him in full mania, raving about hanging his enemies. The reporter thought him quite mad, but many Germans did not. All Hitler's racial fantasies had originated in other minds, generations earlier. Anti-Semitism and a belief in "Aryan" racial superiority were ideas deeply embedded in the national psyche, and the Germans were accustomed to hearing such notions.

"WE SHALL ATTACK"

In the 1920s Hitler gave ample warning that he could not be entrusted with power. He already spoke of war as an end in itself. "We shall attack," he said, "and it is immaterial whether we go ten or one thousand kilometers beyond the present lines. For whatever we gain, it will always be only a starting point for new battles."

Unfortunately, most of those who realized that Hitler's ideas were dangerous thought the man himself was not. Some trusted that the good sense of the German people would keep him from a position of power. Some believed that he did not mean what he said and was merely enlisting right wing support. Some expected that power would sober him or wiser men control him. Many thought Hitler was merely a harmless eccentric because he preferred the role of Bohemian artist to that of politician.

Moreover, Hitler's bizarre behavior, clearly indicative of mental illness, was hidden from most Germans, and most of those who observed his peculiarities did not understand what they meant. His symptoms were interpreted by his retinue as signs of genius; people who were not fellow fanatics were merely mystified. Hitler's conduct at a party he attended in 1923 was characteristic of his weird social behavior and his startling mood changes. A witness reported: "While he was being introduced, he wore the expression of a public prosecutor at an execution. . . ." Hitler spent an hour sitting in silence, eating cake until the hostess made a comment about the Jews. Immediately he stood up, "yelling, in . . . a powerful, penetrating voice," the witness recorded. "After more than half an hour . . . he suddenly broke off." Then Hitler left without saying a word to anyone.

REVOLT AND ARREST

By 1923 the Nazi party was growing and vocal but still small, most of its power and influence centered in a single city, Munich. Nevertheless, Hitler decided that the time had come to start a revolution and to take over all of Germany. The result was the famous Beer Hall Putsch on November 8 of that year. The idea was manic; the outcome was foredoomed not only because the Nazis lacked sufficient power, but also because during the Putsch Hitler slipped abruptly from mania to depression. After giving a fiery speech in Munich's Bürgerbraukeller and shooting his gun at the ceiling like an extra in a Western movie, he muttered, "If it comes out all right, well and good; if not, we'll hang ourselves." He refused to give any more speeches, neglected to order the seizure of vital points in the city, failed to call out his supporting troops, and made no effort to prevent his hostages from escaping the beer hall. At one point he tried to bestow the leadership of the Nazi party on someone else. Hitler became, by turns, apathetic, despairing, and raging. He spent the night walking aimlessly in and out of the beer hall, letting his revolution disintegrate.

The parade Hitler had scheduled for the next day was equally dismal. The government of Munich was still in power and the city police stopped the vanguard of the parade marchers with guns. Several people were shot and killed, including a man who had been walking next to Hitler. The terrified leader ran from the scene and kept going until he found sanctuary in the house of a friend. He informed the lady of the house that he was going to shoot himself, but was prevented from doing so when she wrested his gun from him and threw it into a barrel of flour. Two days later the Munich police found Hitler hiding in the house and arrested him.

The depression continued while Hitler was held in Landsberg Prison, awaiting trial as a revolutionary. For two weeks he refused to eat, citing his belief that the wages of failure are death: "Anyone who has had as great a fiasco as I have had has no right to go on living. . . . I have no other course but death by starvation." A physician who saw the prisoner in January of the following year, noted that Hitler was depressed most of the time, but did have occasional merry moods. Unstable though his moods were, Hitler's paranoid delusions had become fixed, and he expressed them both in his manias and depressions. In that period he wrote, "One can only understand the Jews when one realizes their final purpose: to master the world and then destroy it . . . while they pretend to raise mankind up, actually they contrive to drive mankind to despair, insanity, and destruction." In paranoia, people often project their own darkest motives onto others. Hitler's words were a chilling forecast of his own role in history.

When he came to trial, Hitler faced a sympathetic judge and audience, and took advantage of the occasion to attack his accusers. Propelled by mania, he was confident, aggressive, and eloquent, giving rousing political speeches to applause and cheers. He spent only five months in prison, where, coddled by sympathetic jailors, he lived as if in a hotel. He was allowed visitors at all hours. Many brought the sweet pastries he loved to eat. He was permitted to select a companion, Rudolf Hess, to share his large, sunny cell and serve as his secretary. He felt happy and creative enough to write a book. The result was *Mein Kampf* (*My Struggle*), the terrible manifesto of prejudice and hate that became the Nazi bible.

A MOVEMENT FOR MADMEN

On leaving prison, Hitler fell into a stuporous depression. If he spoke at all, it was after long silences and the words came out at half speed. When his depression wore off, Hitler was able to reconstruct the party that during his incarceration had become demoralized and fragmented. The Nazi party resumed its growth and, within a year, Hitler would win the alliegiance and financial support of a number of Germany's major industrialists.

As the party expanded, Hitler needed assistants. His manic ego required people whose outstanding virtue was their worship of him and their willingness to do anything he asked. His vanity also demanded that he select people with physical or mental handicaps who offered him no competition. Among his acolytes were men with club feet, deformed backs, deafness, missing arms, addictions to drugs and alcohol, and severe mental disorders. They found in Hitler a messiah and worshiped him.

Rudolph Hess, the Nazi party's deputy leader, wrote in all sincerity: "Hitler is like a boy. Riotous, singing, laughing, whistling. . . . Adolf Hitler, I love you because you are both great and simple! A genius!" To Hess Hitler was "witty, humorous, and spirited. He is like a child: kind, good, merciful. Like a cat: cunning, clever, agile. Like a lion: roaring and great and gigantic." Joachim von Ribbentrop, who became Reich Foreign Minister, declared: "It is very difficult to judge a genius like Hitler, for he cannot be measured by ordinary standards. . . . His intelligence was outstanding and his grasp astounding."

Those who managed to contain their enthusiasm did not stay in Hitler's favor very long. Through this trial by sycophancy, he eliminated everyone who was handicapped by intelligence and integrity.

SUCCESS AND SUICIDE

Hitler's rising political fortunes and the largesse of wealthy Germans encouraged a personality change that took place in 1929. He abruptly abandoned the self-denying, Spartan existence of a depressive for the luxurious lifestyle of a manic. He moved from two meagerly furnished rooms to a large, rambling apartment in one of Munich's best neighborhoods. He replaced his modest wardrobe with an expensive and extensive one, and acquired several large new Mercedes automobiles. He also hired twelve servants to take care of his new acquisitions.

Hitler's moods still alternated between mania and crippling depression. He might give five speeches in one day, and then vanish for a week. But speechmaking was usually a powerful antidepressant. At the mass rallies the Nazis organized, the wild excitement of the audience made him manic. At first he would seem nervous and unsure, but soon his voice would increase in volume and his words thunder forth. A witness remembered Hitler "holding the masses and me with them under a hypnotic spell. . . . It was clear that Hitler was feeling the exaltation of the emotional response now surging up toward him . . . his voice rising to passionate climaxes. . . ." Eventually the crowd would reach a pitch of almost religious hysteria. Hitler would finish panting, exhausted, soaked with perspiration. On the rare occasions when he faced an unfriendly or unresponsive audience he could not complete his speech and departed abruptly.

Women could also serve as antidotes to depression. "Women's gushing adulation," one contemporary noted, "carried to the pitch of religious ecstasy, provided the indispensable stimulus that could rouse him from his lethargy."

In the summer of 1931, Hitler's growing grandiosity inspired him to announce: "I intend to set up a thousand-year Reich and anyone who supports me in this battle is a fellow fighter for a unique spiritual—I would almost say divine—creation." It was a manic summer filled with the excitement of campaigning for his party in anticipation of a general election that would, he hoped, pack the German Parliament with Nazis. He was also in love with his niece, Angela Raubel. She had moved into his large apartment and was often at his side during public appearances. By the summer of 1931, however, she could no longer tolerate his constant demands for her presence and obedience.

On September 18, the nineteen-year-old was found dead in Hitler's Munich apartment, shot with his gun. Gregor Strasser, a high Nazi official, reported later that he spent the following three days and nights with Hitler, who confessed to shooting the girl in the heat of a quarrel. Hitler was in a state of extreme agitation, sleepless, constantly pacing, refusing to eat, and Strasser prevented him from committing suicide. According to Strasser's brother, "An inquest was opened at Munich. The public prosecutor . . . wished to charge Hitler with murder, but the Bavarian Minister of Justice stopped the case."

Angela's death was officially attributed to suicide. Whatever the truth, Hitler continued in a severe depression for weeks during which he told people that he would give up politics. He also spoke of killing himself. At this time he became a vegetarian, which he remained for the rest of his life. For many years afterward he kept his niece's room untouched as a shrine to her memory. He also ordered the liquidation of everyone who knew anything about the circumstances of her death.

DEEPER INTO DELUSION

The more closely Hitler approached to power, the stronger his delusions became. This was partly because, as with Napoleon, those around him deferred to his every whim and feared to bring up anything that would trigger his ferocious temper. Dr. Hermann Rauschning, president of the Danzig parliament and one of Hitler's intimates during this decade, said: "I have frequently heard men confess that they are afraid of him. . . . They have the feeling that the man will suddenly spring at them and strangle them, or throw the ink pot at them, or do something senseless."

Hitler grew increasingly isolated from reality. A remarkable glimpse of his anger, delusions, and violent behavior is afforded by an interview with him conducted by Richard Breitung, a German newspaper editor. Breitung's record of the interview includes the following running account. The parentheses are Breitung's.

> (Hitler becomes increasingly irate, bangs his fist on the table and screams) "Don't think I care what the bourgeois press writes about me and my movement! . . ." (Hitler's temper suddenly rose and he became red in the face) "We give orders; they do what they are told! . . ." (Hitler becomes increasingly excited and screams) "If we do not succeed, we shall go to the dogs and we have no wish to go to the dogs. . . ." (Hitler gazes at me and screams) "Do you think I don't know what you're thinking now? You are thinking that I isolate myself, that I refuse to have advisers, that I am not receptive to new ideas, and that I am unapproachable and avoid discussion. . . ." (Hitler becomes more and more excited) "Berlin is no German city today; it is an international muckheap! . . ." (He seemed possessed by a rage for destruction; he was foaming at the mouth, no longer speaking clearly, and so fast that I could not catch his words. . . .)

Incredibly, after this performance Hitler shook hands, walked with Breitung to the door, and said, "I am glad to have had this frank discussion with you. I hope that I have made a real friend." Aware of what his critics had said about him, Hitler—like Napoleon—nevertheless had the manic's insensitivity to the impression he was making as he spoke. Breitung's final conclusion was that Hitler "undoubtedly has a tendency to megalomania," but that in Germany "many people like listening to this megalomania." The editor predicted, "If Hitler comes to power, he will be the end of us all." All three statements were true, and the last became true for Breitung himself when Hitler had him poisoned by the Gestapo.

THE LAST ELECTION IN GERMANY

Having largely recovered from his reaction to Angela's death, Hitler threw himself with wild energy into his 1932 campaign for the presidency of Germany. He went to speak in twenty-one towns in seven days, then on to another twenty-five towns in eight days, and fifty more towns in twenty-four days, traveling often by plane. He was heard by hundreds of thousands of Germans. He lost the election to the incumbent who was a national hero, Field Marshal von Hindenberg. Hitler suffered a post-campaign depression and despaired when Gregor Strasser, one of the pillars of the party, left: "If the party once falls to pieces," Hitler said, "I shall shoot myself without more ado." But he was far closer to success than he realized.

In January of the following year, President von Hindenberg asked Hitler to serve as chancellor of Germany. This offer was made reluctantly, but the Nazi party had become the strongest in the country and the government could not function without Nazi cooperation. Hitler's second-in-command, Hermann Goering, rejoiced: "When the need was greatest the Lord God gave the German people its savior . . . one with overwhelming genius and greatness of character. . . . How seldom are the gifts of genius united with the will to action. In Hitler they find a perfect union."

In November 1933, the Nazis won the elections for the Reichstag with 92 percent of the vote. Henceforth, Germany's government became Hitler's creation. The constitution and all citizens' rights were immediately abolished. State governments were overthrown by storm troopers and taken over by Nazis. Other political parties were no longer permitted to exist. Labor unions were outlawed and replaced by a fraudulent national union. Censorship and the total extinction of free speech were celebrated with great bonfires of books. Germany's prisons filled with those who had openly opposed Hitler; concentration camps would soon swallow the overflow. And the persecution of the Jews had begun with a Nazi-led boycott of all Jewish shops.

THE NEW GERMANS

During Hitler's first three years in power, Germany made astonishing economic strides. Six million unemployed Germans found jobs. The economy boomed; inflation was nil. For none of this, however, was Hitler directly responsible. He achieved Germany's miraculous post-Depression recovery by leaving government to others. Like the artists of the Romantic tradition, he had always ignored financial matters and was not prepared to guide the economic policies of an industrially advanced nation, or any other kind, for that matter. According to architect Albert Speer, who later headed Germany's war production, "He never had a bank account. He did not use a wallet. . . . As a private person he did not know how to handle his own money, and as a head of state he could not manage the government budget."

Germany's economic "miracle" was largely the work of the Minister of Economics, Dr. Hjalmar Schacht, who had begun his restorative work before Hitler occupied the chancellory. Moreover, the German people themselves, with their skills and energy, deserve acknowledgment—they repeated the "miracle" after World War II. Nevertheless, Hitler took the credit for it, as he did for whatever improvements took place in Germany: the superhighways, which he had initially opposed, better factory conditions, free holidays in the country for workers, a lowered crime rate—and the Volkswagen.

Hitler's real accomplishment was to make progress possible by restoring the morale and confidence of the German people. He turned their humiliation to pride, their despair to hope. By imposing a one-party state on Germany, he also quieted the political uproar that had characterized the country through the 1920s. Though pernicious in other respects, this political stability allowed the moribund economy to recover.

The price he exacted was the people's freedom, but most Germans thought at the time that they had made a good bargain, and in their gratitude adored their führer. Foreign political leaders were also impressed with the material progress in Germany. Winston Churchill called Hitler "the greatest statesman in Europe if he preserves the peace of the world."

Foreign visitors who came to see the new Germany found a nation throbbing as though with a single heart. The German people's love for Hitler could not only be seen and heard, but also felt, like the heat of a fever. One of Hitler's interpreters recalled driving in a motorcade with some English and French guests during one of the führer's triumphal processions through Nuremberg. "It was as though at the sight of him mass intoxication had seized untold thousands all along the way. They greeted him with outstretched arms, and shouts of 'Heil!'" The interpreter added that the "Englishmen and Frenchmen [were] moved almost to tears by such scenes, and even some hardboiled journalists were shaken to the core."

A SMALL PURGE

Beneath this shining, benign surface lay a festering world of darkness—the world of the nascent SS, the Gestapo, and the brown-shirted SA Storm Troopers. Hitler had organized the Storm Troopers as a private army in the 1920s to be used whenever it was necessary to destroy political opponents or indeed anyone who aroused his displeasure. Once in power, Hitler no longer needed the rowdy brown shirts, who had become an embarrassment. He used them as a bargaining chip with Germany's military leaders who wanted to eliminate any armed force over which they had no control. Hitler agreed to suppress the Storm Troopers in exchange for military endorsement of his bid to succeed the dying President von Hindenberg. It was also convenient for Hitler to eliminate any possibility of a challenge from the SA's longtime chief, Ernst Rohm. In June 1934, with characteristic ruthlessness, Hitler sent thugs to murder his old friend Rohm. Many other brown shirts who had been early and ardent Hitler supporters were also attacked wtihout warning and killed during "the night of the long knives." Hitler passed off the slaughter as necessary to "halt the spread of the revolt." He did not, he told the Reichstag, prosecute Rohm and the other "offenders" in regular courts because the threat was too great. "In this hour, I was responsible for the fate of the German people, and thereby I became the supreme judge of the German people."

Having thus appointed himself both judge and executioner and gotten away with it, Hitler suffered little anxiety over the murders of his opponents. Among the victims was General Kurt von Schleicher, a former chancellor who had advised von Hindenberg to keep Hitler from power. Hitler also ordered the liquidation of Gregor Strasser, who had left the Nazi party and who knew too much about Angela Raubel's death.

The murder of Rohm was not without its psychological repercussions. For days afterward, Hitler was stricken by a severe agitated depression. He was unable to sleep but refused to take sleeping pills for fear of being poisoned. His paroxysms of crying, vomiting, and trembling seemed to corroborate the delusion that he *had* been poisoned. At times, fearful of the dark, he demanded to have all the lights on. Solitude also frightened him and he insisted that people keep him company during his insomnia. When paranoia increased its hold on Hitler, he sent everyone away, fearful that someone would attack him. This interval of deep psychosis was still in progress when President von Hindenberg died. On that date, August 1, 1934, Hitler added the office of president to that of chancellor and acquired unlimited power over the government of Germany.

THE "INNER VOICE"

The führer suffered from two considerable handicaps as a head of state: he was irrational a good part of the time; and when he was not, he avoided work as much as possible. Hitler craved power, but government did not interest him and he refused to learn anything about it. In only two areas did he concern himself with details; foreign policy and the armed forces. Otherwise, as Albert Speer reported, "he trusted in his inspirations no matter how inherently contradictory they might be. . . ." Or as the führer himself declared, "One must listen to an inner voice and believe in one's fate." When it came to governing Germany, Hitler would give vague orders. Others had to work out the means to fulfill them.

As chancellor Hitler retained the lifestyle of the bohemian artist he fancied himself. He generally rose around noon, took meals at odd hours, was late for most appointments, or did not keep them at all. Historian Oswald Spengler complained: "He cannot work." Hitler also refused to face problems. Dr. Hermann Rauschning, president of the Danzig senate observed, "when difficulties arose, he simply pushed aside everything he had just planned and lost all interest in the pile of wreckage that remained behind."

OBSESSED BY THE ARTS

Hitler said that had the First World War not come about, he would "probably have become one of the foremost architects, if not the formost architect of Germany." But he was not an artist distracted by politics, he was a dictator dilettante. Hitler surrounded himself with artistic failures like himself. Joseph Goebbels, the Minister of Propaganda and Public Enlightenment, was a failed novelist; Alfred Rosenberg, head of the Foreign Political Office of the Nazi party, was an unsuccessful architect. Hitler applied what he thought were artistic standards to everything, including weapons of war. Generals should also be artistic, Hitler thought. When he began World War II, he was willing that the army draft scientists and technicians and send them to the front, but he exempted the musicians of the Berlin Philharmonic.

As with all other matters, Hitler's ideas about the arts were rigid and he refused to learn from anyone. For artists who displeased him, he had nothing but hatred. "If some self-styled artists submits trash for the Munich exhibit," he said, "then he is either a swindler, in which case he should be put in prison; or he is a madman, in which case he should be put in an asylum; or he is a degenerate, in which case he must be sent to a concentration camp." Abstract painters, he added, would be sterilized. Hitler declared that his government was a "dictatorship of genius." Actually it was a dictatorship over genius, which resulted in a diaspora of the best minds and most inventive artists in Germany.

7

"The Greatest German of All Time"

HITLER IGNITES WORLD WAR II

The two previous chapters have described the course of Hitler's manic depressive illness during his childhood and early years in Linz, Vienna, and Munich. These chapters also traced the rise to high office of a man who seemed too deranged for a political career. Nevertheless, having made Germany the most militarized and aggressive nation in Europe, Hitler went on to achieve hegemony over a vast empire. Two questions arise at this point: Why did the Germans accept Hitler as a leader, and why did other European leaders wait so long to oppose so dangerous a man on so obviously destructive a path?

To begin with the first question—why the educated citizenry of an advanced and supposedly civilized nation such as Germany became enthusiastic followers of a madman—part of the answer is, of course, that most of the German people did not know about Hitler's violent mood swings and frothing-at-the-mouth rages. Even those who witnessed his bizarre behaviors did not realized these were symptoms of mental illness. Historian Carl Jacob Burchhardt observed that among the Nazis, Hitler's "frenzied raging, with a total loss of self-control, was considered masculine."

Another part of the explanation of Hitler's popularity lies in Germany's historical situation—the agonizing humiliation of defeat in World War I, a subsequent siege of economic chaos that pauperized the middle class, and a faction-rent government that inspired no confidence. The Germans were accustomed to autocracy and many felt that democracy had delivered the nation to disaster. Hitler's promise of order—and his strong opposition to communism—had enormous appeal to conservative groups, including many clergymen, educators, civil servants, military officers, and industrialists.

He also appeared to the lower classes who sensed that Hitler, a failure during the formative years of his life, was the Teutonic little man, troubled by the same fears and yearnings as his fellow citizens. To the young, Hitler was a hero offering them a purpose in life—the greatness of Germany. To others he appeared as a father offering what Germans had learned to value most in life: security. A follower of Hitler said: "Why do the Germans love Hitler? Because with Adolf Hitler they feel safe!" Moreover, many Germans who voted Hitler into power expected him to be sobered by the responsibilities of government, to forget his wilder promises, and to mature into the traditional leader they desired.

There was also a darker side to Hitler's appeal for Germans—his anti-Semitism. He frequently assured the German people that they had someone to blame for all their misfortune, someone to hate and destroy: the Jew. Finally, as the post-colonial experience of several African nations have shown, when a stable regime has ended and no single person or fraction has legitimacy in the eyes of the people, the winner of the ensuing Darwinian free-for-all is likely to be the least fit for leadership—the most aggressive, power-mad, ruthless contender. Hitler was all of these, thanks to his demonic mania. "I have not come into this world to make men better," he said, "but to make use of their weaknesses."

The second question—why European leaders waited so long to resist Hitler's aggression—has great immediate relevance because many of the same mistakes were made with Saddam Hussein. First of all, Hitler's rearming of Germany, though it violated the Treaty of Versailles, was acceptable to those who wanted Germany to become a stronger bulwark against the Communist menace to the East. Similarly, Saddam's arms buildup was widely approved because Iraq was seen as a counterforce to Syrian ambitions and Iranian fanaticism. Unfortunately, one cannot rely on people who are unbalanced to maintain a balance of power.

Second, in 1936, when Hitler made his first aggressive move by occupying the Rhineland which the Treaty of Versailles had demilitarized, the people of Europe were still traumatized by World War I and the democracies wanted to avoid another war at almost any cost. Consequently, although Hitler had revealed his obsession with pan-Germanist expansion and *Lebensraum* ("living space") in *Mein Kampf,* people believed his protestations that he wanted peace. Although six of his generals plotted to confine Hitler to an asylum before he invaded Czechoslovakia, they were refused essential support from England and France. Hitler's initial conquests—Austria, Czechoslovakia, and part of Lithuania—were bloodless and therefore tolerated by the rest of Europe, Winston Churchill being one of the few who warned, "We are in the midst of a disaster of the first magnitude." Hitler explained that he had only reclaimed what was originally part of Germany and he wanted nothing more, a performance that was repeated when Saddam claimed Kuwait as the nineteenth province of Iraq. When Hitler demanded the Polish corridor, only the Poles were willing to fight to defend that narrow strip of territory. Like an eerie echo, some Americans, remembering the agonies of the Vietnam War, responded to the invasion of Kuwait with signs asking, "Is Kuwait Worth Dying For?"

The fundamental error made with both dictators is based on a misconception of mental illness. The layman's notion is that one is either wholly rational or wholly irrational, but such is never the case. Even Hitler could reason clearly, as he demonstrated with his Machiavellian manipulation of Britain's Prime Minister, Neville Chamberlain. Foreign leaders aware only of Hitler's political acumen assumed that he was therefore a reasonable human being who would respond appropriately to reasonable argument. They failed to understand that though Hitler was logical, his premises were delusional and *unalterable* and, therefore, his conclusions were insane.

Starting World War II was obviously an act of insanity, but the blame for it belongs to Hitler. Or to be precise, by invading Poland, Hitler turned what had been a Japanese plan of conquest of the Pacific theater into a world war. Mussolini's role was peripheral. He was not consulted about the invasion of Poland, and *in toto* Italy conquered only two small countries. Moreover, Hitler decided to begin the conqest of Europe despite the misgivings of his foreign minister and Germany's military leaders. In November 1937, on a sudden impulse, Hitler summoned them to a meeting in his office where, in a manic mood of exaltation, he spoke for four hours, the gist being that Germany would be at war within a year. Hitler's goals were two: to incorporate all German-speaking territories (the former Hapsburg Empire) into Germany and to obtain *Lebensraum* in Poland and the Soviet Union. Neither idea was original with Hitler when he voiced them in *Mein Kampf*. What he contributed now was the manic delusion of omnipotence. "For me," he proclaimed, "the word 'impossible' does not exist." He also chose the timing of the war. Depression had made him a hypochondriac. Even in his manic periods he retained the delusion that he had not much time left. In 1937 he was convinced that he was dying of heart disease. Thus, both manic and depressive delusions contributed to Hitler's decision to declare war, which he announced at a meeting called on a manic impulse.

Hitler prepared for his insane project in a rational way. By mid-1939, he had built the greatest armed force in the world. But he remained delusional and announced: "I am the greatest German of all time." Another irrational element—hatred—formed part of Hitler's determination to conquer Poland. He declared: "If the slightest incident occurs I will smash the Poles without warning, so that not a trace of Poland will ever be found. I'll smash them like lightning with the full power of a mechanized army." He invaded Poland in September 1939, and England, which had just made a treaty of alliance with Poland, declared war on Germany. This surprised Hitler, who had expected England to ignore the treaty and look after its own best interests.

On hearing what England had done, the führer exploded into a rage that was witnessed by a Swedish businessman, Birger Dahlerus. Dahlerus was trying to promote a peaceful settlement between England and Germany. "He grew more excited," Dahlerus recalled,

> and began to wave his arms as he shouted in my face, "If England wants to fight for two years, I shall fight for two years. . . ." He paused and then yelled, his voice rising to a shrill scream and his arms milling wildly: "If England wants to fight for three years, I shall fight for three years. . . ." The movements of his body began to follow those of his arms, and when he finally bellowed: "And if necessary, I will fight for ten years!" he brandished his fist and bent down so that it nearly touched the floor.

The German armed forces defeated Poland in 1939, and that year German generals again plotted but failed to kidnap their führer. The generals were better at leading armies. By early 1941, they had conquered Denmark, Norway, Holland, Belgium, Luxembourg, France, Yugoslavia, and Greece. Only England remained unoccupied and defiant. It seemed that the Germans were well-nigh invincible. These spectacular victories would have overjoyed a more normal head of state, but Hitler's unstable brain chemistry was an invincible enemy, generating spells of anxiety, confusion, and rage. In his baseless fury, he frequently screamed at his generals, thus confirming their impression that he was a lunatic.

DESTROYED BY DELUSIONS

What might ultimately have saved the world from suffering even longer and more grievously from Hitler were the same factors that launched him into war—delusions colored by mania and paranoia. Specifically, what brought about his downfall, as it had Napoleon's, was his attack on Russia. The huge German lunge into the Soviet Union subjected that nation's people to one of the most terrible trials in all history. But it also proved a fatal agony for the German army and air force.

Knowing that Germany lacked the manpower and resources to conquer England and Russia simultaneously, Hitler had intended to annihilate them in sequence. He had long planned to enslave the Russian people and colonize their fertile lands, but not with belligerent forces at his back. England had to be crushed first. For the present, he was safe. He had a treaty with Russia under which Stalin, in the grip of his own delusions, was sending war materiel into Germany. However, paranoia led Hitler to invade Russia while England remained undefeated. He was possessed by paranoid visions of (nonexistent)

Kremlin Jews sending hordes of Russian soldiers to invade Germany. Thus he felt compelled to hurry his own armies eastward. In reality, Stalin was anxious to remain at peace. He did not feel that the Soviet armed forces would be ready to resist Germany for at least another year. Nevertheless, it is not uncommon for a paranoid ruler to launch an offensive, such as Hitler did, against an unsuspecting victim in the belief that he is merely defending himself against imminent attack.

Hitler was also operating under manic delusions of invincibility when he ordered the German forces to begin crossing the Russian border on June 22, 1941. He expected his soldiers to be in Leningrad in three weeks, and boasted that the war would be won before the summer was over. Intoxicated by the same boundless confidence that had deceived Napoleon, Hitler made another of Napoleon's mistakes: sending his armies into Russia without winter clothing or supplies for cold weather. "Hitler actually knew nothing about his enemies and even refused to use the information that was available to him," Albert Speer commented. "Instead, he trusted to his inspirations, . . . and these inspirations were governed by extreme contempt for and underestimation of the enemy."

When winter did come and victory did not, mania gave way to depression. To jolt himself out of his depressive lethargies, the führer began taking amphetamines orally and by injection. By the spring of 1942, multiplying setbacks were plunging Hitler deeper into psychosis. As Speer observed, "Between the spring of 1942 and the summer of 1943, he sometimes spoke despondently. But then, a curious transformation seemed to take place in him. Even in desperate situations he displayed confidence in ultimate victory. . . . [T]he more inexorably events moved toward catastrope, the more . . . he became . . . rigidly convinced that everything he decided on was right." He denied the disasters his armies were suffering in North Africa and Russia. Hitler seemed to have entered some world of his own in which there were only victories and no defeats. Despite his denials, the recurrent crises increased his depression. He was indecisive, his speech hesitant. Impulsiveness, distraction, and confusion grew worse as Hitler's paranoia and delusions expanded in scope. Rages came more often.

Within months of attacking Russia, Hitler's delusions of omniscience inspired him to emulate Napoleon again in assuming the leadership of his armies. But unlike Bonaparte, he had no military training and no experience of war except as an army private. The results, as General Franz Halder, chief of the German General Staff, reported, were disastrous: ". . . [H]is decisions had ceased to have anything in common with the principles of strategy and operations as they had been recognized for generations past. They were the product of a violent nature following its momentary impulses, a nature which acknowledged no bounds to possibility."

Hitler suffered from another deadly defect as a military commander: his foremost concern was his own glory. "Extraordinary geniuses," he said, "permit of no consideration for ordinary mankind." In his contempt for human life, Hitler cared nothing about the casualties among his own soldiers that resulted from his orders. He declared: "That's what the young men are there for." Glory was incompatible with retreat; consequently, Hitler would only order his troops to move forward, like a tank with no reverse gear. Dr. Otto Dietrich, now part of the Propaganda Ministry, attested, "Since he was unable to yield in anything, the thought of moving back, of withdrawing . . . was unendurable." The refusal to allow retreat caused, in addition to other bloody defeats, the catastrophe at Stalingrad where more than a quarter million German troops were surrounded and annihilated. For that matter, Hitler thought that those who were not victorious dishonored him and deserved death. He became enraged when generals surrendered instead of committing suicide. One of his greatest generals, Erwin Rommel, would be given the choice of committing suicide or being executed and having his family persecuted.

The bloodless conquest of Austria had given Hitler four weeks of manic euphoria; when his forces seized Czechoslovakia, he said to his secretaries, "Children, I'm so happy, I'd really like to stand on my head!" But when reports of victory stopped coming, Hitler's cheery enthusiasm evaporated. "Once the possibilities for taking the offensive vanished," Dietrich recorded, "the fire of his spirit went out." The resulting depressions increased Hitler's self-isolation. Dietrich noted that "in the days of his successes Hitler had often gone to visit the troops, to inspire them and strengthen their morale by his presence. However, after the disasters began, he visited the fighting troops only a single time."

Moreover, the führer frequently refused to believe information that was brought to him if it did not please him. When an officer told Hitler some of the discouraging facts about Russian strength, General Halder recorded, Hitler ". . . flew at him with clenched fists and foam in the corners of his mouth and forbade the reading of such idiotic twaddle." On hearing from Halder himself that Russian tank production was running between 600 and 700 tanks monthly, Hitler banged his fist on the table screaming it was not possible because, "The Russians are dead!"

As he had done during his youth, Hitler continued to employ denial and paranoia as defenses against disappointment. Whenever his General Staff officers tried to tell him what was happening at the front, he called them "cowards," "liars," and "idiots." Every difficulty or failure that he could not deny he blamed on treachery. "All generals lie," he insisted. "All generals are faithless." Hitler quarreled with more than half of his field marshals and all of the chiefs of staff, as well as most of his sector commanders. Regardless of the circumstances, he dismissed those who lost battles. This was hardly the best way to sustain the morale of the men he depended on to win his war.

The Hitler whose manic speeches had cast a spell over Germany lost his charisma and his credibility after his fortunes turned. On the rare occasions when he came "into contact with the populace," Speer observed, "his magnetic power over them seemed . . . to have fled." Even Hitler's fanatical entourage was becoming disillusioned and no longer interpreted his erratic moods as signs of genius. Several of the people closest to him, including Field Marshal Hermann Goering and Minister of the Interior Heinrich Himmler, thought that he had lost his mind but did not know what to do about it. In 1942, several generals again made ineffectual plans to lock the führer up as a lunatic.

Hitler was manic again during the last four or five months of 1942, but depression held sway from January to March of 1943. Then he complained that he found humanity so wicked, he often wondered if it was "worthwhile to go on living." He took ineffectual medication for his depression every two days. As news from the various war fronts worsened, depression made Hitler more and more a recluse in his "Wolf's Lair" headquarters in East Prussia. He rarely made speeches and never visited a bombed city. For several months he took meals alone. Propaganda Minister Josef Goebbels and Albert Speer both noted additional symptoms of depression, including a crippling inability to make decisions. Speer observed that Hitler "would appear absent-minded. . . . [H]e suffered from spells of mental torpor and was permanently caustic and irritable."

Hitler would try to escape the reality of the war by refusing to speak of it unless it was unavoidable. According to Goebbels, "He just can't bear the sight of generals any longer." But none of Hitler's evasions, denials, and rages could change the facts that the Germans surrendered at Stalingrad, a quarter of a million of his soldiers surrendered in Tunisia, British and American anti-submarine patrols were chewing up his U-boat fleet, and German cities were being leveled by Allied bombs.

For a time, Hitler's delusions of victory deserted him and left him stranded in reality. He found it unendurable. Speer noted, "When he considered the torments he now had to endure, he would say gloomily, death could only mean a release for him." Hitler almost got his wish. An assassination attempt was planned by officers who had survived the slaughter in Russia and were convinced of the führer's insanity. But the bomb they placed in a brandy bottle on Hitler's plane failed to explode.

By May 1943, the German forces were about to surrender in Africa but Hitler became manic (with occasional oscillations into depression). In autumn, depression set in. Hitler felt lonely and sorry for himself, saying: "Speer, one of these days I'll have only two friends left, Fräulein Braun and my dog." By now his physician, Dr. Theodor Morell, dared to say publicly that the führer was suffering from manic depression.

SAVED FOR SUICIDE

It was becoming clear to many German officers that Hitler was the army's worst enemy. "Once again it was Hitler," Speer observed, "who, in spite of all the tactical mistakes of the Allies, ordained those very moves which helped the enemy air offensive in 1944 achieve success." Moreover, Hitler seemed determined to lead his nation to complete destruction rather than accept defeat. His delusions had indeed set him on that path. According to Speer, that summer Hitler "held to his theory that all the ground that had been lost in the West would be quickly reconquered." When Hitler felt discouraged, he took comfort from the Romantic myth that geniuses always encounter great difficulties before they triumph. Consequently, he prolonged the war, expecting some miracle to bring him ultimate triumph.

The last and most nearly successful attempt by German officers to save their country from Hitler was made in July 1944. A time bomb was brought to a meeting with Hitler. Although others were badly hurt or killed, the explosion only wounded the führer. Immediately afterward, Hitler had a screaming fit for half an hour, but he emerged from the event believing even more firmly in his destiny to conquer the world. His surviving relatively unscathed was proof to him that he was invincible. "Providence has frustrated all attempts against me," he said. "That can only have one historical meaning, that it has elected me to lead the German people . . . not to final defeat but to victory."

After the assassination attempt Hitler had a number of the generals and other officers who had been part of the conspiracy hanged by the SS. This grisly event was recorded on motion picture film in full color. Hitler enjoyed watching the movie and ordered that it be shown to the soldiers of the German army. It was not, however, very popular.

When the Allies entered Paris on August 25, Hitler became depressed again. Now he looked back at the assassination attempt as a missed opportunity: "If my life had come to an end, then for me personally . . . it would have merely been a liberation from worries, sleepless nights, and grave nervous disease." He had suicidal thoughts and discussed both these and his disordered digestion with his generals.

As the American, British, and Russian armies tightened the noose around Germany, Hitler continued to zigzag between mania and depression. Because he happened to be in a manic phase, Hitler was euphoric when the dreaded Russian armies crossed Germany's eastern border in January 1945. In full retreat from reality, he refused to look at photographs Speer had taken to assess the bombed remnants of Germany's industrial plant. But the less Hitler wanted to know, the more he wanted to control. "Hitler was now determining the movement of companies," noted Vice Chancellor Franz von Papen, "and any deviation from his orders was punishable by death. Corps commanders were being forced to sacrifice whole divisions because they were not permitted to order a retreat. The armies in the Saar positions were left to be surrounded when they could have been brought back across the Rhine and used to form a new line." Paranoia convinced Hitler that anyone ordering a retreat must be in the pay of the Russians and should be "killed on the spot, no matter what rank he may hold."

As they saw their world collapsing, many of the people close to Hitler succumbed for a while to his delusion that he was destined to emerge victorious, that something would occur to defeat the enemy. Speer retained his objectivity, but "the departure from reality," he noted, "was spreading like a contagion." Speer, too, finally joined the ranks of would-be assassins and planned to flood Hitler's bunker with poison gas. The plan had to be abandoned when Hitler took preventive measures.

THE COMMANDER OF PHANTOMS

As the end approached, however, Hitler was alone in his delusions. According to Speer, "Everyone would listen to him in silence when, in the long since hopeless situation, he continued to commit nonexistent divisions or to order units supplied by planes that could no longer fly for lack of fuel . . . no one said a word when he more and more took flight from reality and entered his world of fantasy. . . ." The death of President Roosevelt in April of 1945 lifted Hitler into mania again. This was what he had been waiting for—the miraculous event that would save Germany from defeat. Mania also persuaded him that the Russians would soon give up fighting. He could see it all—the English prisoners of war held in Germany would volunteer to fight against the Russians and England, and America would ask for his help in defeating the Soviet Union.

But before the month was over, Hitler was depressed once more and lamented, "Nothing remains. Every wrong has already been done me." But mania would visit him again, instilling him with irrational confidence. While the Russians were shelling Berlin at close range, he remarked, "When I get this thing solved, we must see to it that we get back those oil fields."

The Russians entered Berlin on April 21 and even Hitler could no longer deny that Germany was losing the war. He did not blame himself for anything, but, like Napoleon, decided that his nation had not been up to conquering the world. Unlike Napoleon, however, he sought revenge against his people. Hitler ordered that "the entire leadership of the Luftwaffe is to be hanged immediately." He also gave orders to kill all wounded German soldiers who could not recover enough to fight again. Finally he decided that everything in Germany had to be destroyed. "Not a German stock of wheat is to be left to feed the enemy, not a German mouth to give him information, not a hand to offer him help. He is to find . . . nothing but death, annihilation, and hatred."

This was not an exercise in rhetoric. Hitler specifically ordered that "all industrial plants, all important electrical facilities, water works, gas works, food stores, and clothing stores; all bridges, all railway and communications installations, all waterways, all ships, all freight cars, all locomotives" were to be destroyed. His list also included farm animals and such nonmilitary assets as hospitals, art galleries, churches, nursery schools, and family pets. He gave two reasons for his decision to annihilate Germany: ". . . [T]his nation will have proved the weaker one," and ". . . those who remain after the battle are only the inferior ones, for the good ones have been killed."

Hitler's last days were a condensation of his previous manic depressive existence. His moods changed hourly, in a manner reminiscent of Napoleon after his defeat at Waterloo. Appropriate despair alternated with incongruous euphoria. The führer remained in the grip of his anti-Semitic paranoia. The Jews still worried him and he declared, "If they are not stopped they will destroy us." They were the mirror in which he saw his own evil.

On April 30, 1945, Adolf Hitler's life came to an end in a double suicide in his bunker far under the earth of besieged Berlin. Eva Braun Hitler, his wife of one day, took poison. Hitler shot himself with the gun he always carried.

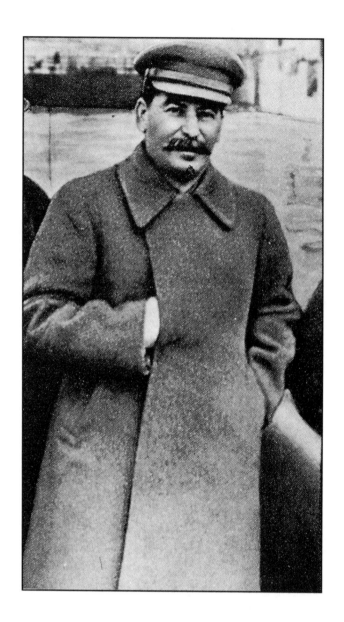

Novosti

Part Three

Joseph Stalin

8

The Red Tsar of Russia

Joseph Stalin was not, like the two dictators already studied in this volume, driven by his delusions to prosecute huge, expansionist wars. His field of destructive action was primarily within his own country, the USSR. There, however, he warred incessantly against his own people, and every group among them: political leaders, soldiers, workers, peasants, and ordinary citizens of every stripe. George Kennan, one of the most perceptive U.S. ambassadors to Russia during Stalin's years of rule, understood this fundamental fact: "The Russian people and the Russian Communist party were as much his adversaries as . . . the world of capitalism." Stalin was, in fact, the world's most destructive anti-Communist, doing more to harm his own nation and its government than any outside force. In these murderous internal campaigns he was driven by the same mental illness that afflicted Napoleon and Hitler. And as with them, his manic depression turned him into a grandiose, merciless tyrant.

Stalin was born on December 21, 1879, into what could be called a tainted family. The place of birth for Josif Vissarionovich Djugashvili, Stalin's real name, was a two-room house in Gori, a village perched among the Caucasus mountains in Georgia, an independent nation until Russia engulfed it early in the nineteenth century. Stalin's father, Vissarion, was unstable, alcoholic, and violent, just like the son who was to rule the Soviet Union. A cobbler by trade, he could not keep a job or make a living—the police listed him as a "tramp"—and he left his family when his son, the only survivor of four children, was four years old. Djugashvili's brief returns home ended in drunken rages, with beatings for his wife and child. Once the boy, trying to stop an attack on his mother, threw a knife at him. Vissarion died at the age of thirty-eight, stabbed in the back during a drunken brawl. He was buried in a pauper's grave. His son was eleven.

Stalin's mother, Ekaterina, a woman of some spirit, worked as a maid and laundress to support herself and her son. She resisted her alcoholic husband's determination to make their child, who was nicknamed Soso, a shoemaker. She had higher ambitions for her boy and insisted that he become a priest. As Soso was growing up, his mother apparently had episodes of mental illness, for she would run disheveled down the streets of Gori, talking to herself, praying, or singing. Either one of Stalin's parents could have provided the genes for his manic deprssion.

THE MAKING OF A REVOLUTIONARY

The boy called Soso early showed facets of both a depressive and a manic personality. The depressive Soso was serious, solitary, shy, studious, and loved reading. The other Soso was described by fellow students as "ordinarily very brisk, mobile, and vivacious" despite a deformed foot and partially crippled left arm. He was also violent, breaking windows, stoning chickens to death, and stealing from his neighbors. He started free-for-alls, fought anyone who disagreed with him, sneered at the troubles of others, and never cried over his own. This manic Soso was rebellious, aggressive, and virtually uncontrollable in school, where he tormented his teachers.

Despite his delinquent behavior, the boy won a scholarship to the theological seminary in Tiflis, which he entered at age thirteen. At the seminary his personality was remarkably like that of Napoleon and Hitler when they were young. Much of the time he was depressed, remaining unsociable and irritable for weeks at a time. He was also egotistical and domineering. He flared up when anyone contradicted him and hit people for jokes that he took as insults. He became enraged when any other student tried to shine in class discussions. Throughout his life Stalin would attack whatever or whomever seemed to have more power than he did. The short, slight youth dominated his schoolmates through what one described as their "fear of his crude anger and his vicious mockery."

Stalin's personality seems to have been set by the time he had reached his last year in the seminary. He had lost his religious faith, and rebelled against the authority of his teachers. "You know, they are fooling us," he told his classmates. "There is no God." It was the seminary, Stalin once said, that led him to his profession. "In protest against the outrageous regime and the Jesuitical methods prevalent at the seminary, I was ready to become, and actually did become, a revolutionary. . . ."

It was at the seminary that Stalin also first tried out some of the political techniques he would later perfect. One was to pursue power for himself by fragmenting any group he entered. He did this with a small secret cell for Marxist students. He split the group, taking with him the members who seemed totally submissive to his leadership. "He deemed it something unnatural that any other fellow student might be a leader," one schoolmate noted. In addition, Stalin shortly won his spurs as a traitor to his friends. Expelled from the seminary, he wrote to the rector accusing several of his fellow students of being, like himself, "politically unreliable." They were expelled as well.

The seminary also taught him thought control. Many books and newspapers were forbidden and surveillance was constant. Ecclesiastics, he later wrote, were adept at "spying, prying, worming their way into pupils' souls and outraging their feelings"—which is not a bad description of Stalin's own method later on.

Lastly, the seminary confirmed and sharpened Stalin's paranoid tendencies and deepened his hatreds. These traits, combined with his manic drive for supremacy and his depressive fear of people, made Stalin into the tyrant he became. "Nothing was added to his character" after the seminary years, according to his daughter Svetlana. The only difference was that later his "basic traits had developed to the utmost degree."

BETRAYAL AND EXILE

Stalin began his career as a professional revolutionary in the city of Tiflis. There he quietly tried to undermine the local party chiefs and gain control. It did not work this time, the party leaders deciding "to exclude him from the Tiflis organization for slander and unprincipled intriguing." This setback had no chastening effect, however, and Stalin continued to divide and conquer whenever the opportunity arose. He early developed another habit as a revolutionary, that of inciting workers to violence and betraying them to the police. A bloody riot that he organized in Tiflis for May Day 1901 filled him with manic excitement. Stalin talked about it so volubly afterward that a friend concluded, "The blood that had flowed during the demonstration had intoxicated him."

Having worn out his welcome in Tiflis, Stalin next went to Batum, a blue-collar town, where he again recruited his own followers and tried to overthrow the local revolutionary leadership. He called the Batum leaders cowards and betrayers of the workers. In 1902, he organized another outbreak of mass violence and told the 2,000 demonstrators, "The soldiers won't shoot us. Don't be afraid of the officers. Just go on and hit them right on the head, and our comrades will be freed." Fifteen demonstrators were shot to death and 54 wounded. A suspiciously timely arrest was all that kept Stalin from being condemned by the Batum revolutionaries as an agent provocateur. A verdict of guilty sent him on his first trip to Siberia.

The following year, after his return, Stalin married Ekaterina Svanidze (Kato)—like him, the child of a cobbler. Their only child, Yakov, was born seven months later.

Since Batum's revolutionaries wanted nothing to do with him, Stalin moved on to Baku, an oil industry center. In his relentless drive for power, he tried to dislodge another revolutionary leader. After the man's arrest, Stalin would have been tried by the Baku revolutionaries as an informer had he not again conveniently been arrested.

While in the Baku prison he spread false rumors that two inmates were police spies. One of his victims was nearly beaten to death by the prisoners and the other was fatally stabbed. Stalin also incited his fellow prisoners to stage demonstrations for which they were punished. He took no part. He had so little feeling for others that he would calmly study German or go to sleep as men were being led past him to the gallows.

The manic Stalin briefly appeared at a conference of Russian Communists in Stockholm in 1906. His roommate described a transformation in the dour revolutionary: ". . . [H]e had astonishingly shining eyes, and he was a bundle of energy, gay and full of life."

In 1907, Stalin buried Kato, who had died of pneumonia. He sent their son to live with her relatives and began a period of criminal activity on behalf of the Bolsheviks, becoming the party's fund raiser in his native Caucasus. He and several professional criminals organized a protection racket, drawing up lists of industrialists, bankers, and shopkeepers and demanding contributions. Those who refused or contacted the police were severely beaten, their families threatened, and their places of work heavily damaged. A man who had police records in two countries was chosen by Stalin to help him run a chain of brothels. Nikolai Lenin, founder of the Bolshevik party, objected to this type of entrepreneurship.

On June 26, 1907, Stalin organized the bombing of a Tiflis bank. More than fifty people, including customers and passersby, were killed. He was expelled from the Bolshevik party and his fellow revolutionaries ordered him again to leave Tiflis. Many of those who knew Stalin in the period between 1901 and 1909 thought he was in the pay of the tsar's secret police. There were too many hasty releases from jail, and quick escapes from exile. His punishments were usually far lighter than those given to his fellow revolutionaries.

During the next years Stalin oscillated between periods of manic activity and morose depression. In 1909, he worked furiously to undermine Lenin's leadership, writing unsigned articles that accused Lenin of what he himself was trying to do—split the party. During a subsequent period of depression, Stalin dropped from sight so effectively that some of his fellow Georgians believed he had abandoned the cause and taken a job in a Baku oil refinery. Elevation to the Bolshevik Central Committee brought a return of manic good spirits—Stalin entertained the family he was living with by doing imitations and telling jokes—but depression returned with a 1913 sentence to further exile. On arrival in Siberia, Stalin remained solitary and uncommunicative; he went directly to his room, refusing to join his welcoming party. On the rare occasions he saw his fellow revolutionaries, he quarreled with them. For the most part, Stalin preferred to spend his days alone in the snowy wilderness, fishing and trapping. In fact, he behaved so disagreebly toward his fellow exiles that after the Russian Revolution freed all the political prisoners, they recommended he not be given an active role in party affairs.

A TASTE OF POWER

This general dislike did not stop Stalin's drive to power. Back in Petrograd in March 1917, he worked with manic energy, soon taking over the party newspaper, *Pravda*. He spent sociable hours with an old friend and fellow revolutionary, Sergei Alliluyev, who had two young daughters, Anna and Nadya. Anna recalled that Stalin smiled often that April and would bring food for the family suppers. Over glasses of tea, he entertained the girls with tales of his Siberian exile, readings from Russian classics, or doing imitations of people he had recently met.

Depression returned in the fall of 1917, although by then the Bolsheviks were in power and Stalin had been named the Commissar for Nationalities. The excitement of the civil war that soon gripped Russia shook him out of his lethargy, however. So did a new assignment from Lenin to go to Tsaritsyn as Director General of Food Supplies for the South of Russia, and to make sure enough grain reached Moscow.

Stalin tackled his new job with murderous energy. Even before leaving for Tsaritsyn, he sent orders ahead: ". . . [B]e absolutely ruthless. A number of villages should be set on fire and burned to the ground." But once on the scene, Stalin did little about the grain shipments. Instead he began a wholesale purge of the local military leaders, accusing them of sabotage and having them executed—a performance he would repeat on a nationwide scale twenty years later. Stalin replaced the murdered officers with men of little experience and limited ability such as Kliment Voroshilov, a friend from the Baku days. Their distinguishing qualification was that they obeyed his orders instead of those coming from their superior, Leon Trotsky, the creator and commander-in-chief of the Red Army.

Throughout his career, Stalin would, like other egotistical and dominating manics, promote those he could control absolutely over those who were competent but less malleable. It was a costly policy. After Stalin left Tsaritsyn, Lenin complained that "60,000 Red Army men were lost because of Stalin and Voroshilov." Nevertheless, Stalin cherished the grandiose belief that his work at Tsaritsyn saved the Revolution.

Stalin also took over command of the city, putting his own men in charge of the government offices and looking everywhere for supposed conspirators. Entire families were executed without trial as traitors. Tsaritsyn, in fact, was a preview of the way Stalin would take over the Soviet Union: substitution of his own adherents in the civilian and military seats of power, with illegal arrests and executions of all possible opposition. Throughout, Stalin betrayed the symptoms of mania that Trotsky later pinpointed: "ferocious energy and enterprise" combined with a "passionate self-assurance which one day grew into a conviction of his political and military infallibility."

Paranoia also clearly played its part. Stalin instituted another practice he was to employ throughout World War II: ordering the execution as "traitors" of Red Army soldiers who had been captured by the enemy. As Trotsky observed, "a military setback or a strategy of which he did not approve became in his mind products not of error or accident, but of treason." This twisted, paranoid interpretation of reality would become the rule during Stalin's years as dictator.

Despite his realization that Stalin was unreliable at best, Lenin kept giving him tasks to perform—perhaps because he thought Stalin too uneducatd to be a serious rival. In January 1919, Lenin sent Stalin to Perm to investigate a surrender there of the Red Army. Predictably, Stalin repeated the Tsaritsyn pattern, executing whomever he chose and putting his own men in command. In May, Stalin was in Petrograd, supposedly to save the threatened city. Impelled by his mania and paranoia, Stalin accused the Soviet General Staff of being enemy agents and executed 67 officers who disagreed with his military decisions. He was at last recalled to Moscow while Trotsky himself took charge in saving Petrograd from capture.

Between these episodes, Stalin chalked up some successes, gaining several positions of power at the March 1919, Eighth Party Congress. He also remarried. During an earlier manic period, the forty-year-old Stalin had managed to charm and seduce the sixteen-year-old Nadya Alliluyeva. Her father insisted he marry the girl, who was already pregnant.

But there were more setbacks to come. Stalin was rebuked by the Politburo for military failure—and then suffered an additional defeat in mid-1920 when he was sent to be military commissar on the southern front. Stalin's dreams of military glory were fading fast and he fell into a depression. He lost interest in the war, which, in any case, was winding down. The speeches he gave were listless. That November he was rushed to a Moscow hospital for an emergency appendectomy. While convalescing, Stalin planned to take revenge on his native Georgia, which, against his wishes, had been recognized as an indepedent state. He would order the Red Army to "cauterize" the opposition "with red-hot irons."

TAKING OVER, INCH BY INCH

Depression was, in fact, dominant in Stalin's personality—at least while Lenin lived and ruled. In his brief manic periods Stalin had intense productive energy, made impulsive decisions, and could be ingratiating or explode in anger. When depression prevailed, he was sulky and indolent, avoided meeetings, and kept to himself for days. At such times he was indecisive, cautious, and silent. But not even depression diminished Stalin's obsession with power. Unobtrusively, he gathered the reins of government in his hands.

In 1920 Lenin gave him control of the Orgburo, which determined all admissions to, explusions from, and promotions within the Communist party. This was the sort of position the wily Stalin understood perfectly how to use. "A country is in fact governed," he said, "by those who have really mastered the . . . apparatus of the state." This was true enough in the centralized, bureaucratic Soviet Union. Given control of the right governmental levers, a man with no popular appeal, with no army behind him, could seize the highest office.

Lenin never intended that it should happen. When he allowed Stalin to become General Secretary of the Central Committee in 1922, it did not appear to be a position of great potential. But then Lenin suffered his first stroke, and while he lay stricken by partial paralysis, Stalin began to fill the political vacuum. Within months Lenin realized that Stalin had "concentrated limitless power in his hands."

Despite Stalin's clever maneuvering, one of his rages nearly destroyed his future in the party. He had tapped Lenin's phone and overheard Lenin's wife, Nadezhda Krupskaya, talking with Stalin's chief competitor, Trotsky. They were planning to unite against him. Stalin telephoned Nadezhda and cursed her, threatening to expel her from the party. He ordered her to stop all discussion of politics and party matters with Lenin, and threatened to try her before his Central Control Commission. He screamed, used obscene language, and called her a whore.

Nadezhda told her husband the threats Stalin had made. Lenin dictated a letter to Stalin saying: "I have no intention of forgetting what was done against me, and it goes without saying that what was done against my wife I also consider as having been directed against myself." He insisted that Stalin apologize or face "the break-off of relations between us." Lenin could, at that point, have expelled Stalin from history.

In fact, he tried, but the effort came too late. In January 1923, after his second stroke, Lenin wrote a political testament rejecting Stalin as General Secretary. "I propose to the comrades to find a way to remove Stalin from that position and appoint to it another man who in all respects differs from Stalin in superior qualities—namely, more patient, more loyal, more polite; and more attentive to other comrades, less capricious, etc." Unfortunately, the document was not released and Stalin later suppressed it.

As Lenin faded, he became ever more convinced that Stalin was treacherous. "He lacks," Lenin said, "the most elementary human loyalty." Stalin doubtless got wind of all this and may, to save his own political skin, have hurried Lenin to his grave. Stalin had assumed the responsibility for Lenin's medical care and he told Trostky and other Politburo members that Lenin had asked him for poison to avoid a lingering death. Actually, the invalid's condition was improving at the time. Lenin died shortly thereafter, on January 21, 1924, with a suddenness his physicians did not expect and could not account for. Stalin sent Lenin's widow a poisoned cake for her birthday fourteen years later, obliterating her name from Soviet history books after her demise. He also demonstrated his veneration for Lenin by killing all those who had, before the Revolution, given Lenin refuge, gotten him out of prison, helped him return to Russia, and protected him from the tsar's police.

Lenin's death, natural or not, saved Stalin from public disgrace and left the Georgian poised to take over the Soviet Union—provided he could eliminate the others who jostled for supremacy. Preaching unity, Stalin leaped deftly from one side to the other, always landing with the majority, while his rivals attacked each other. By December 1927, Stalin had performed considerable surgery on the party: seventy-five members of the opposition had been expelled from the Party Congress and many others were already in prison. Two years later Trotsky, who had seemed Lenin's most likely successor, was deported, to be murdered some years later by an agent Stalin sent to Mexico. Then Stalin diposed of his remaining competitors, Gregory Zinoviev, Nikolai Bukharin, and the others. "The miraculous Georgian," as Lenin had called him in better days, would continue keeping his associates isolated and weakened by their envy and fear of each other—a strategy that would make Stalin's overthrow impossible and allow him to pick off his victims at will.

MANIC FULFILLMENT

In the mid-1920s, as Stalin destroyed his opposition and tightened his grip on the USSR, the manic, expansive side of his personality came to the fore. He gave noisy parties, and his daughter Svetlana recalled the period as the brightest of her childhood. "The colorful Semyon Budyonny [one of Stalin's military puppets] would bring his accordion and play Russian and Ukrainian songs. My father would sing, too," she added. "I still have pictures of happy summer picnics on which they'd all go." In his manic phase Stalin liked to bowl and play billiards, and kept his house filled with the in-laws whom he would later kill at the bidding of his paranoia.

Mania had an aphrodisiac effect on Stalin. He shocked even his male friends with his gutter language and obscene songs. He became so promiscuous that in 1926, Nadya took her son Vasily and six-month-old Svetlana to her parents' home in Leningrad. Stalin insisted they return. The next year she threatened to commit suicide if he did not break off his affair with a singer.

Stalin drank more as the tension of his marriage increased and his drunken behavior became insupportable. On one occasion he drunkenly brought a secretary to Nadya's bed, waking his wife and telling her that he wanted to compare the two women's sexual techniques. Nadya ran screaming into her daughter's bedroom and locked the door. An infuriated Stalin smashed his wife's photograph and spent the night with the secretary.

In 1929, the year he turned fifty, Stalin's behavior was ruled by his manic ego. The cautious, modest-seeming, depressive politician had been transformed by absolute power into a manic tyrant who acted as though he were a god and demanded to be worshiped as the USSR's Supreme Pontiff, the sole interpreter of Marxist-Leninist Holy Writ. He tried to extend his dominion over time itself, rewriting the history of the Russian Revolution so that it was "he who had organized the Bolshevik party, led the October Revolution, commanded the Red Army, and had been victor of the Civil War and the wars outside Russia." Stalin also assumed credit for the work of Lenin, Trotsky, and Zinoviev in running the Comintern, which organized Communist activities abroad. Miraculously, Stalin, who had nearly been court-martialed twice for disastrous defeats during the Civil War, emerged as the sole hero of both the Revolution and the Civil War.

Stalin's New Testament, *The Short Course of the History of the All-Union Communist Party,* appeared in 1938 to become the only acceptable version of the recent past. People who had copies of the document in which Lenin recommended removing Stalin from power disappeared into prisons or graves.

The almighty Stalin could modify the past of others as easily as he did his own. He removed Trotsky's name from all official histories; the Red Army was forbidden to mention its founder's name when celebrating its anniversaries. Everything already in print was amended to conform to the new Gospel. The Institute of History, on Stalin's orders, fired all members who refused to follow the Stalinist line. Old comrades who refused to revise their memoirs in accordance with the new myth were liquidated. "His hatred of us," one of these doomed heretics said, "is motivated chiefly by the fact that we know too much about him."

A MODEL FOR STALIN

Stalin chose as his *beau idéal* Ivan IV, or Ivan the Terrible (1533–1584), the first of Russia's rulers to assume the title of "Tsar." Stalin so admired his forerunner that he ordered a film made about Ivan to depict him, in Stalin's words, as "a great and wise ruler." Stalin's only criticism of Ivan was that the tsar's liquidations had not been sufficiently complete. Stalin's secret police were consciously modeled on those of Ivan.

In this tsar, Stalin found a paranoid, grandiose, manic depressive who shared his taste for seeing the blood of others shed, although Ivan, living in a more primitive age, had more freedom to indulge in torture as an entertainment. Russia of that day, in fact, was a cavalcade of violence. A contemporary English visitor, shocked by Russian brutality, wrote: ". . . 'Ere the sun dawns in Russia, flagellation begins; and throughout its vast empire cudgels are going . . . from morning until night." Ivan's boyhood amusements included dropping dogs from high towers to see them splatter on the street. As ruler, he had peasant women kidnapped, stripped, and released in his palace courtyard so that he could watch his men shoot them as they tried to escape. His rages were even more violent than those of Stalin, and when angered, Ivan would strike whoever was within range of whatever weapon he happened to be holding at the time. He would smash furniture and dash his head against the floor. In a fit of anger Ivan killed his own son by striking him on the head with a staff.

In his most severe depressions, such as those following the deaths of his son and his first wife, Ivan pulled out hair from his beard and his head and banged his head against the wall, only to emerge from his depression raving about his suffering and covered with blood. He threatened to commit mayhem against himself, as well as against others, and claimed repeatedly that he would give up the throne to enter a monastery. Unlike Stalin, Ivan felt remorse during his depressions, spending days in prayer, making confessions of guilt, and uttering pleas to God for forgiveness. During his later years he passed increasing numbers of days in silence, refusing to see anyone; or he would creep around abjectly, complaining of his martyrdom and obsessing about his fear of God's anger. Ivan had the pusillanimity of many depressives, especially when it came to personal danger. Despite the calls of his generals, who awaited his leadership, he refused to emerge from his tent until a battle was over.

Ivan's manic periods were apparently more intense, or at least less restrained, than those of Stalin. When manic, the tsar was utterly driven and incapable of rest. He was overbearing, and became, as he himself admitted, "a stinking dog living in drunkenness, adultery, murder and brigandage." Ivan encouraged his fellow Russians to drink because the treasury profited thereby. Even then, alcoholism was a national problem. An English visitor noted: ". . . To drink drunk is an ordinary occurrence with them every day in the week."

Like Stalin, Ivan was most manic at night, which often was spent in drunken banquets with his cronies, when he sang, danced, and played occasionally lethal practical jokes. These parties, unlike Stalin's, were often enlivened by mass sexual orgies and exhibitions in which bears killed prisoners. During periods of Ivan's life he had women captured to provide him with new flesh daily. He also kept a harem of some sixty women and girls. Like Stalin, Ivan had the manic's love of the gigantic and grandiose: he designated himself as God's special agent. Ivan also established his own cult of personality, and from his day forward, the tsars expected and received a worship second only to that of God.

Ivan's grandiosity contributed to his paranoia. He once punished a noble for addressing him without proper respect by having the man's tongue cut out. Like Stalin, Ivan reduced the likelihood of revenge against him by annihilating entire families, including their sympathisers. Years of proven loyalty to Ivan were often rewarded by imprisonment and torture. Ivan's paranoia extended even to visiting ambassadors and other foreigners, who were constantly supervised wherever they went and confined to living in a special part of Moscow.

Ivan equated surrender with treason. He also anticipated Stalin by executing government personnel and army men of high rank for the disastrous effects of his own cowardice, when by fleeing Moscow he left it undefended, to be burned and looted by the Tatars, who took 100,000 captives as slaves.

Bizarrely enough, after all the horrors of his reign, Ivan was mourned, like Stalin, at his death by the entire nation, including the children of his victims.

PRAISED BE THE LORD

As Stalin consolidated his power, the fever of adulation for him rose steadily. The Party Congress of 1930 said very little about Stalin's achievements. The Congress of 1934 spoke of little else. No speaker dared to omit elaborate flattery at each mention of the General Secretary's name. The national anthem that Stalin approved praised him alone, omitting any reference to the Communist party. Trotsky noted that Stalin "had to have the press extol him extravagantly every day, publish his portraits, refer to him on the slightest pretext, print his name in large type. Today even telegraph clerks know that they must not accept a telegram addressed to Stalin in which he is not called the father of the people, or the great teacher, or genius. The novel, the opera, the cinema, paintings, sculpture, even agricultural exhibitions—everything has to revolve around Stalin as around its axis."

Epithets for Stalin abounded. He was the "Man of Steel"; "the Brasshard Leninist"; "the Soldier of Iron"; and, as a change from metallurgical metaphors, "the Bolshevik of Granite." He also enjoyed terms Hitler favored: "Universal Genius" and "Greatest Genius of All Times and All Peoples." Many thousands of farms, schools, factories, businesses, barracks, power stations, towns, and cities were also given Stalin's name.

The Georgian was a jealous god. Churches and temples were pulled down by the hundreds, and monasteries disbanded. Priests and even hermits were imprisoned, deported, or killed. Icons, sacred books, and religious objects of every kind were destroyed; religious schools were closed and proselytism forbidden. Stalin tried to eliminate any allegiance other than to himself. Husbands, wives, and children were exhorted to place loyalty to Stalin above love for family.

Nikita Khrushchev noted that the Soviets saw Stalin as "a superman possessing supernatural characteristics, akin to those of a god. Such a man supposedly knows everything, sees everything, thinks for everyone, can do anything, is infallible." This is precisely what a manic in the grip of his psychotic delusions believes about himself. Stalin once admitted: "I have never met my equal."

For the tyrant, no adulation is excessive. *Pravda* published the suggestion that a new calendar be instituted substituting Stalin's birthday for that of Christ, and making 1879 the new year "One." The Georgian enjoyed hymns if they were in praise of himself and commanded that these be sung daily at theaters, stadiums, circuses, and in the streets. Even those children whose relatives had disappeared into the prisons and camps had to recite with the rest, "Thank you, dear Stalin, for our happy childhood."

9

The First Soviet Holocaust

To make his war against the Russian people, Stalin first had to fight the Communist party, get it under his complete control, and convert it into a weapon. This he began to do in the mid-1920s. As usual, Stalin preached the opposite of what he was doing, making comforting remarks about keeping the party intact. "An amputation policy is full of dangers," he said in 1925. "Today one is amputated, another tomorrow, a third the day after. What will be left of the party in the end?" Two years after he made these reassuring comments, Stalin expelled 3,258 members from the party, including seventy-five of the most prominent. Many of those expelled were deported or imprisoned. Three years later, Stalin ejected another 130,000, more than 10 percent of the party membership. By 1928, then, no significant opposition remained at any level in the party and Stalin was free to run the USSR according to his desires.

A MANIC FIVE-YEAR PLAN

Like many leaders of developing countries, Stalin was in a hurry to industrialize. He began by robbing Soviet citizens to finance his industrialization. Beginning in 1928, anyone suspected of owning precious metals, gems, or foreign currency was arrested; interrogated nonstop; screamed at and threatened; deprived of food and sleep; beaten; and held captive until madness, death, or the payment of sufficient ransom ended the torture.

As he advanced from a position of political dominance to one of absolute power, between 1926 and 1928, mania invaded Stalin's policies and view of reality. When a Five-Year Plan was drawn up for the entire Soviet economy, Stalin set goals that were ridiculously optimistic. In 1928, the first year of the plan, it was clear that the production targets were too high. But by then Stalin believed in his omnipotence. As he put it, "There are no fortresses which we Bolsheviks cannot storm and seize." The next year, without explaining where the money would come from, he quadrupled the funds to be spent on industrialization.

By 1931, Stalin's manic extravagance and grandiosity inspired him to order the construction of gigantic, unworkable farms, factories, and other construction projects. Lack of funds kept many of them uncompleted for years while others had to be abandoned altogether. Manic delusions kept Stalin from seeing that his production quotas and grandiose projects were unachievable. That year several economists were tried and imprisoned for setting production targets that he felt were too low. Although even their modest targets were not met, Stalin had by then deluded himself into believing that the USSR was already surpassing the major industrialized nations of the world: "Relatively little is left for us to do," he insisted.

THE SECRET CIVIL WAR

Another of Stalin's manic delusions was that he could transform Soviet agriculture overnight. When reality thwarted his will, his obstinacy and vengeance resulted in the first Soviet holocaust. It all began in the fall of 1927, when many of Russia's peasants, expecting a price rise, withheld grain from the market. The following January the dictator sent Red Army troops into the villages to seize the harvest. A witness recalled that they "went from house to house, day after day, looking for hidden food. . . . Sometimes whole walls were pulled down. . . . Peasants were hauled to headquarters and there subject to all-night interrogations, beatings . . . and semi-naked confinement in cold cells."

What began in 1927 developed into a lopsided civil war. On one side were the Soviet farmers; on the other were Stalin and the Red Army. The farmers reduced their production, slowed deliveries, and hid their harvests. Stalin sent the Red Army into the countryside. Resistant villages were surrounded with machine guns; soldiers shot randomly at the residents. Sometimes all the people living in a village were hanged. Farmers rioted and attacked government officials. The most fertile provinces were depopulated, their fields abandoned to the wind and weeds.

Stalin announced a campaign of extermination: "We now have the opportunity to mount a decisive offensive against the kulaks, to break their resistance, to liquidate them as a class." He characterized the kulaks as a small group of wealthy farmers, but suddenly kulaks were everywhere. Anyone who resisted collectivization or expressed opposition to it, any person who voiced sympathy for "kulaks," became a kulak himself. Instant kulaks were created by neighbors who accused those against whom they held grudges, or whose property they coveted.

In rebellion against Stalin's harsh measures, the peasants began to slaughter their animals rather than surrender them to the state. In six years, horses, cattle, and pigs were reduced to about half their former number, sheep to one third, and the total agricultural capacity of the USSR diminished to three-fourths of what it had been. Determined to take vengeance on the only segment of the Soviet population that had attempted to defend itself against him, Stalin decreed long prison terms for any infraction of the rules, such as small thefts of grain. In one year alone, three million "kulaks" and their families were deported to Siberia; millions more were shot or sent to prison camps. Some were condemned by quick tribunals, while others were simply eliminated by the secret police.

By 1930, more than half of the farmers in the Soviet Union had been forced into collective farms. Within three years, 125 million peasants had become, in all essentials, serfs of the Soviet Unoin and its dictator. Stalin's serfs were told what, when, and how much to plant, to raise, to harvest. They were told where to live and work. To make matters worse, they were not paid enough for what they produced, Stalin being determined to finance the industrialization of the USSR with the profits from agriculture—whether there were any profits or not.

STALIN'S FAMINE

In a fatal oversight, the dictator's plan for 1928–1933 neglected to provide enough barns for storage of the harvest and enough vehicles to bring it to the mills, which also were insufficient. Consequently, much of the harvest was lost. Stalin guaranteed that the following years would also be disasters by insisting that quotas be met regardless. Thus many collective farms had to surrender the seed for the next year's crop plus their own food supplies and that of their animals.

Paranoia protected Stalin's ego by casting blame elsewhere. At first it was the "kulaks" who had sabotaged his plans. Now it was the collective farmers who, Stalin insisted, were hoarding grain. Even collectives that somehow met their quotas were guilty—of hoarding a surplus. Furthermore, kulak saboteurs were still at work in the collective farms, busily pretending to cooperate. A new crime was invented: "connivance in or toleration of pseudo-cooperation." Blame even attached to party officials, who were arrested for failing to seize the grain that Stalin imagined the starving peasants had hidden. In 1933 almost three dozen people had been executed without trial for such forms of sabotage as having "allowed weeds to grow in the fields."

Dogs and cats, rats, and mice were killed for food. In some villages, the desperate turned to cannibalism. "Entire villages perished, including children and old people," Soviet historian Anton Antonov-Ovseyenko recorded. "Those that had strength to move headed for the railway stations and the towns, paving the roads with their corpses."

In the cities food rations were reduced to near-starvation levels. Thousands, suffering already from severe malnutrition, were felled by dysentery and typhus. Factory workers died at their machines. In the morning, wagons cleared the streets of the skeletal, frozen corpses and dumped the bodies into mass graves. As for the children who survived, Stalin instructed the secret police that those caught stealing food must be killed immediately. Homeless orphans were clogging railway stations by the thousands that year. Stalin's order significantly reduced the problem.

During Stalin's onslaughts against the farmers, the Soviet standard of living, already reduced by years of revolution and civil war, fell to two-thirds of its previous low level. This did not deter Stalin, who wanted exports to pay for foreign machinery that he needed to rush industrialization. The worldwide depression had ruined the grain market, but he paid no attention. Stalin's will must prevail even over world economics. In 1931 he exported more than 50 times as much grain as he had in 1928, although the crop that year was 12 percent below normal.

The grain exported that year would have saved more than four million lives in the Soviet Union, but Stalin the omniscient denied that there was any famine. According to Soviet statistics released after the dictator's death, he drove some five million people from their homes and farms, and exiled them to desolate areas where only the hardy and fortunate survived. A total of 22 million died either from his persecutions and executions during collectivization, or in the famine that resulted from his disruption of Soviet agricuture and his exports of food. This, the first of Stalin's three holocausts, exceeded Hitler's holocaust of the Jews by some 16 million people.

Of the extent of the disaster Stalin remained resolutely ignorant. He made the last trip of his life into the countryside to observe agricultural conditions in 1928. Even then he avoided the farms, limiting his visit to three towns where he told the party secretaries that the time had come for drastic measures. From that point on, Khrushchev reported, Stalin refused even to talk to farmers and "knew the country and agriculture only from films. And these films had dressed up and beautified the existing situation. . . . Many films so pictured Kolkhoz [government farm] life that the tables were bending from the weight of turkeys and geese. . . . Stalin thought it was actually so."

More than the movies, it was Stalin's manic delusion of infallibility that convinced him his agricultural policy was a triumph and the famine of 1932–1933 a fiction. In 1932, when a party leader from the Ukraine begged Stalin for famine relief food shipments, he replied: "You made up a story about

hunger, you mean to frighten us, but nothing doing. You had better leave
. . . and go to work for the Writers' Union; you will write fables and morons
might read them." Stalin was furthered in his delusions by Soviet statisticians
who had learned to stay alive by telling him what he wanted to hear.

CITY SERFS

In 1930 Stalin inaugurated his campaign against the Soviet worker. A new
law discontinued unemployment relief; it also decreed Draconian punishment
for negligence, for any kind of damage to machines or materials, and for vio-
lations of labor regulations. As of 1932 workers were, in effect, Stalin's property.
They could not legally quit their jobs or be rehired without the government's
permission, while the government retained the power to draft them into factories
and move them from one job or location to another against their will. People
were instantly fired for missing one day of work. Theft of property owned
by the state or by collectives became a capital crime and large numbers of
executions immediately commenced. With these laws Stalin held the Soviet
worker in a death grip that did not loosen during the dictator's life. At the
same time, the tyrant was clamping totalitarian controls on the peasantry, who
constituted the majority of the Soviet population. The Soviet Union had thus
become a nation of captives.

SUICIDE STALIN-STYLE

During the winter of 1932, the level of marital conflict rose in the Stalin home.
Nadya accurately accused her husband of "blood purges and liquidations."
On one occasion she shouted, "You are a tormentor, that's what you are!
You torment your own son . . . you torment your wife . . . you torment the
whole Russian people!" He yelled, "Shut up, damn you!," grabbed her by
the neck and shook her.

   Having decided to leave her husband, Nadya made plans to move to her
sister's home in Kharkov and get a job, but she did not live long enough
to make her escape. The night of her death she left a dinner in a rage because
Stalin had insisted that she drink. He stayed on without her. Nadya did not
go directly home, but arrived at her apartment around 1:00 A.M. Not long
after she got there, she told the governess, Trushina: "Until now I've been
a sort of wife to him, but not any more. I'm nothing. The only prospect is
death. I shall be poisoned or killed in some pre-arranged "accident." Where
can I go? What can I do?" The two existing stories of Nadya's death agree
that Stalin was telephoned, and that he returned from the dinner.

   According to Trushina's version, she found Nadya lying dead on the bathroom floor with a large wound in her temple and a blood-stained revolver on the floor near her. Trushina carried Nadya to her bed and applied a bandage to the wound, although it appeared to be too late to do any good. Before the governess could telephone for a doctor, an aide of Stalin's appeared and forbade her to call anyone, saying, "We don't need any doctors here." Three more of Stalin's inner circle soon arrived, joining him in his bedroom, while Trushina stayed in Nadya's bedroom with the corpse.

The following morning, Abel Yenukidze, one of the men who had spent the night in Stalin's room with the new widower, emerged and asked Trushina if anyone else had seen or heard anything. When she said no, he answered "Good," and told her to explain to the children that their mother had died a natural death. Yenukidze helped Trushina to make the body as presentable as possible, applying cold cream and powder to the young woman's face and covering the wound with her dark hair.

Before the children woke, Yenukidze ordered the governess to pack immediately for a few days "rest." She never saw the children again and was soon in prison. The doctor who signed the death certificate was liquidated, as was Yenukidze, who had been Stalin's friend and best man at the marriage now tragically terminated.

Svetlana's nurse told a different story: Nadya was found in the morning on the floor of her bedroom with a small pistol in her hand. The nurse and the governess cleaned the body and called Stalin's friends, who arrived while Stalin slept through everything.

There is no mention in either account of anyone hearing a gunshot although at least five people—the two children, the nurse, the governess, and Stalin—were present in the apartment when Nadya supposedly shot herself. It seems more likely that Stalin killed her by striking her on the side of the head with the gun. That would explain how a small gun could have produced a large wound and become stained with blood.

Stalin's subsequent behavior followed a pattern that he repeated whenever he had political enemies liquidated. He erased Nadya from the past, removing or killing every person who had witnessed her last years. Her servants and the children's teachers disappeared. Her friends and family were imprisoned and/or killed. He obliterated every physical reminder of his wife's existence. Sveltana noted, "everything which she had created with her own hands and efforts was being systematically destroyed . . . her knickknacks disappeared. All her papers and personal belongings were taken away." Svetlana claimed that Stalin stayed away from the funeral and never visited Nadya's grave.

Svetlana did not see her father during the days following her mother's death, but relatives who were with Stalin said he was in a state of violently fluctuating emotions: when he was not suffering from fits of rage, he spoke of wanting to die. His rage was evident when he went to the public viewing of Nadya's coffin and gave it a quick shove. Three weeks later Stalin was still filled with fury. A speech he delivered was so sulphurous with threats against the peasants that it was not published.

Stalin limited his appearances in public for a while; but by the time four months had passed, he was joking with the First All-Russia Congress of Collective Farm Shock Workers, trying to make them believe his manic fantasies about 20 million poor peasants who had become prosperous from collectivization.

THE BEGINNING OF THE "TERROR"

Stalin's second holocaust commenced on December 1, 1934, with the assassination of Sergei Kirov, who had been designated as a possible successor. Kirov assured Stalin that he had no such ambitions, but realized that it made no difference. "They're going to kill me," Kirov told a friend. After Kirov was shot by Leonid Nikolaev, an unwitting tool of the NKVD (the Soviet secret service), further murders were ordered to deflect suspicion from Stalin. Kirov's bodyguard, Borisov, was beaten to death on the way to his interrogation. Borisov's wife was interrogated about what her husband had told her, then confined to a mental hospital. Though she managed to escape and claimed that a poisoning attempt had been made, she was returned to the hospital where she did indeed die of poison. The men who killed Borisov were shot themselves. A woman who had known Kirov's assassin, her sister, her sister's husband, and everyone who had ever recommended her for a job were imprisoned. Stalin was nothing if not thorough. The dictator then used Kirov's murder as the pretext for a wave of executions in Leningrad, which had been Kirov's power base. Many of those whom Stalin killed as conspirators in Kirov's death were already in prison before the murder took place.

Stalin had already decreed that entire families would be punished for the crimes of individual members. As the terror machine began to roll, attempts to leave the USSR, and even the "intention to leave the country" without government permission, became punishable by death. The minimum age for death penalties was dropped to twelve. By the mid-1930s, the citizens of the Soviet Union had become simultaneously prisoners and hostages. One out of every ten Soviet men had suffered banishment, exile, imprisonment, or execution.

There was a curious pause for about a year while Stalin behaved like a manic campaigning for office. He was everywhere, beaming at festivals, bestowing prizes at athletic competitions, giving out dolls to children, handing out accordions to productive workers, and donating rubles to loyal officials. He posed at workers' banquets with little girls on his lap.

Stalin saturated the entire country with his manic fantasies. An emigré reported, "We read jubilant books, listened to jubilant speeches, and saw jubilant movies. All made essentially the same point: Stalin was the wisest, the kindest, the most courageous, the most omniscient, and the most prescient. He was our Father whose heart swelled with love for us. And the life he created for us, so we were told and eventually believed, was the best of all possible lives." Stalin himself proclaimed, "Life has become better, comrades. Life has become more joyful." For a brief time it was true. Food rationing was ended. Peasants were permitted to keep small plots and a few animals for their own use or profit. Fashion magazines became legal. Factories added manicurists to the staff. The Kremlin became festive with balls and the pop of champagne corks. The Communist party treated the citizens to carnivals, feasts, sports, and dances. Stalin gave the country a new constitution.

But this sunny interval was not to last. Its end, in August 1936, was signaled by the trials of Stalin's former colleagues, Gregory Zinoviev and Lev Kamenev, for the murder of Kirov. The executions of the leaders of the Russian Revolution began with them. Many more trials and killings would follow in what became infamous worldwide as The Great Purge.

10

The Second Soviet Holocaust

RITUAL SLAUGHTER

In 1928 Stalin invented a form of entertainment that would be the most publicized feature of the purge to come. His invention, the "show trial," was given
its first run when eighteen engineers were tried for sabotage and espionage
at the Shakhty coal mines. They were imprisoned and subjected to treatment
that guaranteed they would confess and accuse each other in the courtroom.
Without any additional evidence, their testimony was supposed to prove that,
as Stalin said, "this group of bourgeois experts operated and wrought destruction to our industry on orders from capitalist organizations in the West." This
trial was soon followed by another in which forty-six people were found guilty
of sabotage of the food industry—although members of the secret police later
admitted they could not find a shred of evidence to support the charges.

Stalin's paranoia shielded his ego from recognizing his mistakes. Enemies
became his favorite explanation for all disappointments and failures. He ascribed
everything that went wrong in his industrial Utopia to sabotage, which he
termed "wrecking." Stalin's suspicions were intensified by his jealousy of educated people. Any of his countrymen who had industrial and scientific training were in his mind potential enemy agents. "Bourgeois wrecking," Stalin
proclaimed, "is an indubitable sign that capitalist elements have by no means
laid down their arms, and that they are gathering stength for new attacks
on the Soviet Union."

There was an abundance of blame to spread around during the late 1930s.
The Second Five-Year Plan was not performing any miracles, and the citizens
of the Soviet Union knew that their lives were still hard and hungry. The

show trials provided explanations, however fanciful, for the shortcomings of communism and scapegoats, however innocent, for Stalin's errors and crimes.

Ironically, the show trials broadcast to the world that the USSR was not the workers' paradise Stalin had declared it to be. The confessions placed in the mouths of Stalin's scapegoats were a litany of Soviet failures never before admitted publicly. Successive trials revealed that the collectivized farmers were mistreated, that workers were abused, that industry was inefficient, that consumer goods were inadequate and of poor quality, and that the non-Russian republics seethed with discontent over their treatment by the government in Moscow.

Beginning with the trials of Zinoviev and Kamenev in 1936, show trials were also used to incriminate others for deaths ordered by Stalin. Through the show trials, Stalin disclosed that a number of deaths originally attributed officially to natural causes were homicides. These murders, too, had been committed at his command. However, others paid for them. Henry Yagoda, chief of the secret police, and a number of physicians who signed false death reports were convicted of numerous murders, including the poisonings of the writer Maxim Gorky and his son.

Nikolai Yezhov, who replaced Yagoda as NKVD head, was another who died for Stalin's sins. The story given out was that Yezhov went insane and, having been placed in an asylum, hanged himself from a tree while wearing a placard saying "I am filth." That confessional touch undoubtedly originated with Stalin. Later he forgot that Yezhov was officially a suicide and remarked, "That scoundrel Yezhov! He finished off some of our finest people! He was utterly rotten. . . . That's why we shot him!"

An additional purpose of the show trials was to rally the country against Leon Trotsky, who was in exile, and his followers, who were few. "Trotskyism was completely disarmed," Khrushchev later commented, adding that "there was no basis for mass terror in the country." Nevertheless, though Stalin had controlled the selection of all party members, government officials, and bureaucrats for the previous ten years, his paranoia told him that many of these men were followers of Trotsky or agents of capitalist governments and had to be destroyed.

SOVIET PSYCHODRAMA

Stalin's show trials had several unique features that gave these ceremonies an anachronistic quality more appropriate to the tribunals of the Inquisition than to twentieth-century jurisprudence. One was Stalin's reliance on confession as evidence, which is quite contrary to modern practice. His secret police would have had no difficulty manufacturing physical evidence, but apparently Stalin was not interested in such material.

Another peculiarity of the show trials was that those who confessed often lavished compliments on Stalin while admitting to treason and other crimes. The "confession" of Kamenev included the following, written in Stalin's hand: "The leadership of Stalin is made of too hard a granite to expect it would break apart by itself." Stalin's poetic insertions did not increase the credibility of the confessions. However, the flattery that Stalin extorted from his victims not only satisfied his ego, but also demonstrated the extent of his triumph over them and deepened their humiliation. Stalin designed these dreams to feed his own ego. His need to appear merciful was satisfied by ordering "lenient" sentences of only ten or twenty years—and then having the prisoners killed in the camps by criminals in the pay of the NKVD.

Stalin shared Hitler's delight in cruelty for its own sake. The Georgian sent NKVD agents to Germany to learn Gestapo techniques in 1933 and 1934, well in advance of the purge. Initially Stalin counseled restraint: "Beating people up, torturing them physically and breaking their bones, is all right as far as ordinary peasants are concerned." Later he approved such methods for everyone and some of the "interrogations" went on for months.

Some historians have explained the purge as a rational, though ruthless, elimination of the entire spectrum of opposition. This theory, however, does not explain why Stalin killed his local supporters along with old Bolsheviks who had retired from active life because of infirmity or age, and could no longer pose any sort of threat. It does not explain why he killed people whose only offense was that they were refugees from Nazi Germany, or poets from the Ukraine, or that they complained about the size of the meat ration. Among Stalin's favorite victims were his former comrades, men who had fought the tsar and been exiled to Siberia with him. He destroyed, Soviet historian Roy Medvedev has said, "many old Bolsheviks who were personally devoted to him, never said anything against him, and carried out all his orders." Stalin exterminated any Bolsheviks who deserved admiration and gratitude for their services to the nation. As Medvedev has observed: "He wanted not only unlimited power but also unlimited glory; no one must upstage him in the historical drama." And no one was spared. Even deceased Bolsheviks were declared "enemies of the people." Finally, Stalin banned the word "Bolshevik" from the Soviet Union in 1952.

DECIMATING THE PARTY

After killing off Kirov's supporters, Stalin liquidated most of the members of Seventeenth Party Congress of 1934 because they had expressed a preference for Kirov. The members of the congress had cast nearly 300 votes against Stalin while casting only three votes against Kirov. All except three of the anti-Stalin votes were burned and the election was falsified in Stalin's favor.

Only about two dozen of the 1,961 delegates to the Party Congress escaped Stalin's persecution during the purge.

The dictator's deadly vengeance also struck higher targets. The Central Committee, which met immediately following the Party Congress, did not re-elect Stalin General Secretary, but instead made him only one of four joint secretaries. Some members also voiced objections to the executions of fellow members Bukharin and Rykov. Stalin had 98 of the 139 men in the Central Committee arrested and shot.

Paranoia inspired Stalin to clean house again and again. Although he had been placing his own choices in party positions since 1919, his paranoia allowed the new Stalinists to remain in office only a few days, weeks, or months before they, too, were arrested. The process of installation and liquidation of people sometimes did not stop until the fifth replacement was in office. Under such conditions legal authority and governmental functions throughout the Soviet Union broke down. Between 1934 and 1939, more than two million party members were killed or imprisoned. During 1937 and 1938 alone, more Communists were killed by the NKVD than all those who had perished in the decades of struggle against the tsar, the Revolution, and the ensuing civil war combined. Stalin's answer: "A reasonable amount of distrust is a good basis for collective work."

Stalin was afraid even of those he had vanquished: "Defeated groups," he said, "may revive and stir." The exile he feared most was Trotsky. During the Spanish Civil War, a conflict primarily between Communists and fascists, Stalin sent NKVD agents to Spain to kill any Communists who could possibly be Trotskyites. His fear unassuaged, Stalin later killed many of the NKVD agents, military leaders, and soldiers he had sent to Spain, and also liquidated Spanish refugees seeking asylum in the Soviet Union for fear that they had all been contaminated by pro-Trotsky sentiments. The Georgian tyrant killed more of the Soviet soldiers who had fought in the Spanish Civil War than the fascists themselves had. Among his victims were twenty-two Russians to whom he had awarded medals for heroism.

Even after World War II, Stalin continued to kill Communists of every nationality who had fought against the fascists in the Spanish Civil War. He saw them all as followers of Trotsky although the latter had been dead for several years. For Stalin, an enemy was never dead.

POETIC JUSTICE

In 1936 the NKVD still contained individuals who were concerned with law enforcement. One of these, Drovyanikov of the Leningrad NKVD, told a meeting of colleagues: "Comrades, we are not uncovering conspiracies, we are fabricating them. We are persecuting and killing people on the basis of unfounded and slanderous charges." Drovyanikov was executed. One NKVD agent did not wait, and shot himself after writing, "I can no longer take part in the murder of innocent people and the fabrication of spurious cases."

By the end of 1936, those secret police who were insufficiently ruthless were gone, by either suicide or execution. After Stalin had two successive NKVD chiefs killed, he also murdered many higher ranking officers to eliminate the possibility of lingering loyalty to the deceased. As an extra precaution, Stalin liquidated the entire staff of Lefortovo Prison four times over.

The Soviet armed forces and the NKVD had their own espionage services. Stalin annihilated the higher ranks of these agencies and several sets of replacements. The lower levels of all Soviet espionage agencies were also decimated. For paranoids there are never sufficient precautions. Soviet intelligence agents abroad were ordered to return. Some who guessed that execution awaited them disappeared, but they were hunted down all over the world by a special NKVD section created for the purpose. One master spy, Richard Sorge, evaded capture, but his wife, who lived in Moscow, was arrested and killed.

LETHAL XENOPHOBIA

Stalin's war against Communists was not limited to the Russian variety. In 1936 the Central Committee of the Yugoslav Communist party, having been invited to Russia, was annihilated there—with the exception of Tito, who managed to get away safely. The leaders of the Indian, Korean, Latvian, Lithuanian, Estonian, Bulgarian, Czechoslovakian, Hungarian, Romanian, Finnish, and German Communist movements were brought to the USSR and imprisoned or killed. Of some 50,000 Polish Communists in Russia, no more than eighty survived the purge. Italian, Spanish, French, Dutch, Chinese, American, and even Brazilian Communists were imprisoned or killed when they made the mistake of visiting the Soviet Union.

Thousands of Communist refugees who crossed the Soviet border while fleeing fascist and Nazi persecution soon found themselves in Stalin's camps. They had believed his declaration: "According to our Constitution, political emigrés have the right to reside in our territory." He sent German-Jewish Communists back to Germany.

Stalin arrested more members of the Communists' international organization, the Comintern, in a few months of the purge than the rest of the world had done in twenty years. The majority of those foreign Communists who resided in the USSR during the purge died while their comrades in the prisons of capitalist countries survived. The most dangerous place in the world for a Communist of any nationality to be during the purge was the USSR.

Anyone who survived the Soviet government abroad, whether as a member of an international Communist organization or as a Soviet diplomat, was likely to be called home and killed on suspicion of disloyalty. Dozens of ambassadors were liquidated; those who refused to return were killed abroad. Ordinary Soviet citizens who spent any time abroad became prey of Stalin's paranoia. Fifty thousand Soviet citizens who had been employed by the Chinese Eastern Railway when it was partly Soviet-owned were imprisoned as "Japanese spies." Athletes who had gone abroad for competitions were imprisoned. The Red Army band that returned from a 1937 concert in Paris was arrested at the railway station.

Merely to have the slightest contact with foreigners made one an object of suspicion. Numerous stamp collectors were arrested. The woman who brought milk to the German Consul was arrested; so was the veterinarian who treated the German Consul's dogs. The veterinarian's son was also arrested. Two engineers and their families were arrested after receiving from an uncle in Poland a package containing shoes, crayons, and dolls.

THE BEST AND THE BRIGHTEST

Some of Stalin's victims apparently were selected because they aroused his envy. Nikolai Bukharin observed that "he cannot help taking revenge on people, on all people but especially those who are in any way higher or better than he." Bukharin, among the many intellectuals who had looked down on Stalin, joined them in death. Unions of artists and writers were annihilated—in the Ukraine hardly a writer survived. Hundreds of the leading members of educational and scientific groups of every kind throughout the USSR were imprisoned for many years or killed.

Journalists also became Stalin's targets. Having boasted, "You will not find a state anywhere else in the world where the proletariat enjoy so great a liberty of the press as in the USSR," Stalin imposed five layers of censorship and imprisoned or had shot the editorial boards of the major reviews and the staffs of the largest papers, *Pravda* and *Izvestia*.

Stalin, like Hitler and Napoleon, treated his fellow human beings as members of an inferior species—a variety of vermin, with the difference that Stalin dressed his policies in humanitarian pronouncements. "We should cherish human beings," he said, "as carefully and attentively as a gardener cherishes his favorite fruit tree." Like Hitler, Stalin sent people to his camps in unheated freight cars without sanitation facilities, food, water, or room to sit down. And the Soviet labor camps were hardly better than Hitler's death camps. Guards shot prisoners with little provocation. Prisoners who became too weak to work had their rations set below the minimum for survival. On the average, half of the prisoners entering the camps each year were dead two to three years later. Almost all those who entered the prisons and camps in 1936 had perished by 1940. Stalin's camps did not close when Russia entered World

War II. For the last two decades of the tyrant's life, the total camp population stayed at around ten million and at times increased. The rate of mortality remained abominable.

Although Hitler's death camps, with their gas chamber and crematorium efficiency, became better known, the first such camps were established by the Soviets in 1921. Later, Stalin made heavy use of death camps. During the busy years of 1937 and 1938, 50,000 prisoners were "processed" at Bamlag, in Eastern Siberia, alone. Lacking Cyclon B and other German technology, the Soviets tied prisoners together and piled them like logs onto trucks, to be driven to remote areas where they were shot. Permafrost prevented the digging of burial pits, so the corpses were piled into hills and covered with earth. At camps where the climate permitted, corpses were dumped into huge pits, which were then plowed over. When the Soviet death camps were closed, all remaining prisoners were killed, then special NKVD squads liquidated the camp personnel. Knowledge of the locations of the bodies of millions of Soviet citizens vanished; the records of executions were destroyed.

Stalin was a master at erasing the witnesses to and the physical evidence of his crimes. But he went beyond what prudence required and tried to banish his victims from reality itself. He destroyed, insofar as he could, every trace of their ever having existed. Their families and friends disappeared; their possessions were lost; their photographs, letters, and personal effects vanished. Those artists who had left a legacy to humanity had their paintings, poems, novels, and articles destroyed: the work of their hands and minds was removed from the past, the present, and the future.

RESISTING BELIEF

One of the most frightening aspects of the Great Purge was the lack of resistance to it. Most Russians believed Stalin's claim that he was persecuting their enemies. He saw to it that leading citizens in every profession and industry signed statements praising the justice and necessity of the executions of their colleagues. Many of those who thought the purge excessive, believed that Stalin did not know what his underlings were doing. Unlike Hitler, who wrote *Mein Kampf,* outlining his designs to rule the world and kill the Jews, Stalin gave no such warnings. Instead, he made countless humanitarian pronouncements. People could not imagine that he was responsible for the purge, and attributed it to the NKVD chief, Yezhov.

Stalin also managed to keep the visible part of the purge within acceptable boundaries. Very few people knew the real dimensions of what was happening. Most trials were secret and it was illegal to seek any information about them. The NKVD kept many imprisonments and executions hidden even from surviving family members, either by saying the arrested had been transferred or by claiming that the missing had been exiled without the right to send letters. Deaths due to torture were officially attributed to natural causes: murders were disguised as accidents or suicides. Except for the show trials, which were widely publicized, most people heard only of local arrests of those they knew.

Those who suspected that something terrible was happening had only two choices: to face reality and acquiesce in crime, or to believe Stalin's lies. Flight was impossible, and resistance seemed hopeless. A Soviet writer explained: "If you wanted to live, the most convenient way for an unhappy, distraught, but honorable person clinging with his last ounce of strength to his place in society . . . was to believe."

THE MURDER MACHINE

In order to facilitate persecution on a national scale, Stalin changed the laws to speed the process. The victims were given only one day's notice of trial— no time to prepare a defense—and the accused was denied a lawyer and the right even to speak except to confess. It was standard procedure to arrest first and investigate, if at all, later. No appeals for mercy were permitted, no sentences revised, and execution of sentence took place at once. "When it is a question of annihilating the enemy," said Stalin's chief prosecutor, Andrey Vyshinsky, "we can do it just as well without a trial." Often that was the way it was done—sentences decided in advance, needing only Stalin's signature to become final. Wherever trials were held, they were generally modeled after Stalin's show trials, requiring only confessions extracted by torture. The torturers were paid for each confession.

In 1937 Stalin changed the NKVD into an army, including divisions and regiments, at four times its former pay and with many additional special privileges as well. NKVD agents were dispersed throughout the nation, into organizations and institutions of all kinds—factories, farms, and railroad stations. Agents were delegated to watch other agents, and other agents delegated to watch the watchers. Even children were under surveillance: in one town NKVD agents arrested 60 youngsters, none more than twelve years old, as a "terrorist counterrevolutionary group."

The NKVD also organized a nationwide network of stool pigeons, the "seskots." It was not necessary, however, to become a seskot to take advantage of the hysteria and have one's own personal purge. As Khrushchev observed, "In those days it was easy enough to get rid of someone you didn't like. All you had to do was submit a report denouncing him as an enemy of the people; the local party organization would glance at your report, beat its breast in righteous indignation, and have the man taken care of." Historian Medvedev recalled that people denounced others "to get a good job, an apartment or a neighbor's room, or simply to get revenge for an insult." People also denounced friends whom they thought were about to denounce *them*. As the paranoia spread, party members who failed to find sufficient numbers of "enemies of the people" in their areas were censured and became suspect themselves. Ultimately the USSR became a nation of informers. "Wives disavowed their husbands," the writer Ilya Ehrenberg noted, "and resourceful sons heaped abuse on hapless fathers." In one of the first show trials of the early 1930s, a boy of twelve took the witness stand to demand the death sentence for his father. People who were arrested were forced to denounce their friends and members of their families.

"A MASS PSYCHOSIS"

Stalin's paranoia became official during the purge: the USSR was thoroughly infiltrated by traitors. Denunciation was, therefore, the duty of every citizen; it became the equivalent of a loyalty test. Medvedev claims that Stalin created "a mass psychosis." "Millions were poisoned by suspicion. They believed Stalin's story about a ubiquitous underground and were caught up in the spy mania." While Stalin did not literally make people psychotic, he presented his psychotic view of reality through all the sources of information available to the nation, and no other view was permitted expression.

He insisted, moreover, that people either believe or at least act according to his manic delusion that everything in the world he had made was perfect, and that therefore all defects of whatever kind were the work of "wreckers," says Medvedev. "The smallest error of a manager, miscalculation of an engineer, misprint overlooked by an editor or proofreader, . . . was taken to be deliberate wrecking and cause for arrest. . . . Even such difficulties as the low pay of teachers, . . . high dropout rates from high school, the wearing out of equipment, were demagogically attributed to sabotage." Any kind of accident or breakdown sent officials hunting for enemy agents.

But perfect results did not put Stalin's suspicions to rest. He expected the saboteur to be disguised as a model worker. "A real wrecker," he said, "will from time to time do good work, because it is the only way for him to gain confidence [of others] and to continue wrecking." When there is no way to identify the enemy, paranoia can expand indefinitely, and this was the course Stalin's thinking took. Literally everyone became suspect. As with other paranoid dictators, Stalin transformed his country until it became the very nightmare of his delusions.

Stalin's paranoid fear of everyone around him became a rational response to reality for Soviet citizens. Anyone, for any reason, at any time, might be denounced to the NKVD by anyone else. Two pedestrians who met on the street by chance risked being denounced as a conspiracy. Ovseyenko notes,

"Everyone and everything was feared. The neighbors in your building, the caretaker in the building, your own children. People lived in fear of their co-workers, those above them, those beneath them, and those on the same level. They feared oversights or mistakes on the job, but even more they feared being too successful, standing out."

By late 1938, the Great Purge had become unmanageable. NKVD agents had incriminating documents on every leading official in the Soviet Union, and half of the urban population was in their files. An average of one member per every family in the USSR had been arrested. Since each arrest was supposed to uncover additional suspects, it was a mathematical certainty that the purge would run out of victims. Stalin may have realized this, or simply shifted to a brighter mood. In March 1939, he announced, "In the main, socialism has come into being in the USSR." He attributed this to "the complete liquidation of the opposition." He then declared with manic confidence that the capitalist nations were rushing toward disintegration while the Soviet Union had developed a flourishing agriculture and was the world's strongest, greatest industrial power.

By the time Hitler's forces invaded Russia in June 1941, the Soviet Union had been the scene of a campaign of persecution and extermination that far exceeded, in scope and the number of lives lost, Hitler's genocidal policies. As the purge progressed, more than seven million people were executed and nineteen million imprisoned, a majority of whom also died. Stalin's paranoia had annihilated most of the leading members of the government and the Communist party, the elite of the foreign service, the best brains in industry, the universities and the sciences; the nation's most gifted writers and artists; the top ranks of the armed forces and espionage agencies, and the most prominent members of foreign Communist parties.

Not only did Stalin eliminate those who had made the revolution and defended it during the civil war, he eliminated those who were building the country and were responsible for its defense. So terrible was the purge that in March 1938, Mussolini asked if "Stalin could have secretly become a fascist." Mussolini's confusion is understandable: Stalin had become by far the most effective anti-Communist of all time. His paranoia had become a potent fifth column, working for the USSR's enemies. "Russia hardly exists in our calculations today," announced Hitler's foreign minister, Joachim von Ribbentrop, in 1938. "As long as Stalin makes himself as useful as now, we need not particularly worry about him as regards military policy." By the time the USSR was attacked by Germany, the Communists in Stalin's prisons and camps outnumbered all of the Communists in all the prisons in the rest of the world. Stalin had imprisoned or killed millions of Soviet citizens for treason, but it was he who was the real traitor. The man who invented the term "enemy of the people" was the one who had done the most to earn it.

Stalin's paranoid attacks on his countrymen continued throughout the rest of his long rule. They never again, however, reached the same level of frenzy. But other horrors were to come. Stalin had gone far during the purge to destroy his own defense industry. The country was simply not ready when Hitler attacked, and Stalin prevented his armed forces from preparing any sort of defense—he equated defense with defeatism. His criminal "wrecking" contributed, with a good deal of help from Hitler, to the third Soviet Holocaust. And as if that were not devastation enough, Stalin wiped out his military leadership.

11

Stalin's Third Holocaust

DECAPITATING THE ARMED FORCES

Stalin's third Great Purge hit in large measure the Red Army and air force. Since Stalin never forgot or forgave, all the old-time officers who had criticized his military mistakes during the civil war were *ipso facto* disloyal and therefore liquidated or imprisoned. But the purge of the Soviet officer corps went much further than that. Stalin's fear of a military coup sent him on a murderous rampage, wiping out any and all high ranking officers who had enough prestige to become a threat. Before he was done, he had eliminated almost 90 percent of the Soviet Union's top commanders. Another 35,000 officers were also killed or imprisoned, leaving only one out of every two unarrested. Just as it had shattered the government and the party, Stalin's paranoia brought down the armed forces: "The military staff underwent two, three, even four changes of command," Khrushchev attested. "Men who had earlier occupied third- and fourth-rank positions were promoted to the top after those in the first and second ranks were shot." Medvedev noted: "Never did the officer [corps] of any army suffer such great losses in any war as the Soviet Army suffered in time of peace." By the end of the purge, all the experienced commanders were gone and only one-fifth of the remaining regimental commanders had any experience of command.

The waves of slaughter also carried off teachers and students in the military academies along with military men who had retired to civilian life. Thorough as always, Stalin imprisoned his victims' wives, children, and other relatives. After the German invasion, although arrests of military men continued, Stalin had to release several thousand officers to take charge of his leaderless regiments. Khrushchev observed: "There's no question we would have repulsed the fascist invasion much more easily if the upper echelons of the Red Army Command hadn't been wiped out."

While he was physically annihilating his country's military leadership, Stalin did his best to destroy the loyalty of lower ranking men to such officers as he allowed to survive. Members of all of the armed services were required to participate in the national paranoia by denouncing their superiors. Stalin as usual permitted no loyalty to anyone but himself.

CRIPPLING THE DEFENSE INDUSTRY

Stalin's sabotage of his country's military capability was not limited to the armed forces. He also liquidated many of those managing the defense industry, slaughtered the men responsible for the supply of strategic materials, and killed the leading weapons designers. His interference shut down mortar production in 1936. The execution of its designers caused a delay of two years in the production of the "Katyusha" rocket launcher. His arrest of his leading radar technicians launched Russia into the war without radar. The three top rocket experts were imprisoned; many other weapons scientists, inventors, and engineers were killed. Thousands more were arrested. Some survived to be recalled to their work after the German invasion, including one of Russia's most famous physicists, Lev Landau, and the airplane designer Andrei Tupolev. For most, the war came too late.

The manufacture of guns and other weapons was also severely crippled when defense plant administrators, managers, and shop superintendents were removed, in many cases for failing to meet impossible production quotas. One factory director shot himself; everyone who was suspected of having read his suicide note attacking the purge was eliminated. By 1939 very few were left of the people who knew how to run factories that made machinery, and the same was true for the chemical and electrical industries as well as for the nation's railroads. Those who remained to run the economy were largely inexperienced, and worked under conditions of unbearable uncertainty. Any failure to fulfill quotas was treated as sabotage. Workers became terrified of making the slightest mistake because it could cause their arrest for treason. The result was a general slowdown of production. Thus Stalin prepared his country for the onslaught of what was then the best military machine in the world.

EASY TARGETS

Stalin thought to stave off any attack by the Germans at least until 1942 through the notorious pact he had signed with the Nazis in August 1939.

The pact gave him a free hand to invade Estonia, Latvia, Lithuania, and eastern Poland. It also, he thought, offered him an opportunity to conquer Finland, which had refused to cede territory he had demanded. With manic overconfidence, Stalin disregarded the invasion plan prepared by his generals, whom he accused of exaggerating Finnish strength and underestimating Soviet power. So sure was Stalin of his own infallibility that he planned for the war to last only a few days. He sent inadequate forces, neglected to provide reserves, and did not bother to supply his troops with winter clothing or skis.

The result, inevitably, was disaster for the Red Army which, in addition to Stalin's irrational planning, was crippled by a lack of experienced officers. In three months of winter fighting, the Russians suffered casualties, according to official Soviet figures, that outnumbered the entire Finnish army of 200,000. Khrushchev later claimed that Soviet losses actually amounted to a million men. Instead of conquering little Finland, Stalin settled for the slice of territory he had originally demanded and the Finns remained independent.

Nevertheless, Stalin declared, "Let the trumpets of victory sound." The Soviet soldiers returning from Finnish prison camps were greeted with triumphal arches and a banner proclaiming, "The Fatherland Greets Its Heroes." Then they were marched straight to cattle cars that carried them to slave labor camps. When Stalin made mistakes, he always found someone to punish.

KREMLIN FANTASIES

Stalin knew Hitler was untrustworthy, and would sooner or later attack Russia. He convinced himself, however, that he was clever enough to manipulate the führer, forestalling the German invasion by acceding to Hitler's demands until the Soviet Union had managed, now that the purge was over, to reconstitute its armed forces. According to his daughter Svetlana, Stalin "had not guessed or foreseen that the pact of 1939, which he had considered the outcome of his own great cunning, would be broken by an enemy more cunning than himself." Stalin said repeatedly, "So they thought they could fool Stalin? Just look at them, it's Stalin they tried to fool!" Once having decided on a policy, he could not conceive that it might have been mistaken.

Stalin was also relying on the hated capitalist nations to keep Hitler busy. He was pleased when the Germans invaded France, Holland, Belgium, and the Netherlands on May 10, 1940. That, he was confident, should tie up the Nazis for some time to come. His optimism turned to despair when, in a matter of weeks, France caved in and the British retreated across the English Channel. ". . . [I] was with Stalin when we heard about the capitulation of France," Khrushchev recalled. "He let fly with some choice Russian curses and said that now Hitler was sure to beat our brains in." Under the blow,

Khrushchev added, "Stalin's nerves cracked," and he began to worry constantly with good reason about the condition of the Soviet forces and defense industry. There were times, Khrushchev recalled, when Stalin was "paralyzed by his fear of Hitler, like a rabbit in front of a boa constrictor." Khrushchev observed Stalin in subsequent periods of depression when the dictator felt, Khrushchev noted, "as though the walls were closing in on him."

A year later, the Red Army's equipment and spare parts were still inadequate and the defense industry was turning out obsolete tanks, planes, and artillery. The Red Army had fewer rifles than the tsar's army had at the start of World War I. According to Khrushchev, "part of the problem was that Stalin tried to supervise our manufacture of munitions and mechanized equipment all by himself, with the result that no one really knew what state our arsenal was in. . . . For his part, Stalin very much overestimated the preparedness of our army . . . he was under the spell of the films showing our parades and troop maneuvers. He didn't see things as they were in real life. He rarely left Moscow. In fact, he rarely left the Kremlin."

Stalin's paranoia also impeded defense preparations. Although many Soviet divisions were under strength, Stalin kept ten million men of draft age in prison camps, and reserved a force of some three million armed men in the Secret Police to maintain his grip on the USSR.

He also nearly doomed the Red Army through his manic conviction that he was invincible. Consequently, any planning for defensive war was in Stalin's mind tantamount to treason. He executed Soviet intelligence officers who gave him reports about the technological superiority of German weapons. And, because Stalin did not believe in defense in depth, no troops were allocated to back up the front line in case of a German breakthrough. On his orders supply depots were located so close to the frontier that huge quantities of fuel, weapons, and ammunition needed by Soviet forces were within easy reach of the Germans soon after the invasion began. This policy led to the surrender, in the first days of the war, of dozens of Soviet divisions whose supply depots had been overrun.

THE OSTRICH IN THE KREMLIN

Stalin also set his army up for catastrophe through simple irrational denial. By the spring of 1941, German troops had been massing on the Soviet border for months and were arriving in mounting force. Stalin's delusional solution to this threat was to deny that it existed. His paranoid imagination created the notion that some German spies and generals were making a pretense of war preparations to goad him into declaring war. If he refused to respond to their provocations, he could postpone the war until 1942. Feeling secure in his self-deception, he resolutely ignored all contrary evidence.

Growing numbers of German spies were caught on Soviet territory. German planes increased reconnaissance flights over the USSR. German deserters and Soviet frontier troops reported the massive German buildup on the border. Stalin ignored all this, as he did warnings from both Winston Churchill and the American State Department that war was imminent. The top Soviet spy, Richard Sorge, reported from Tokyo the precise date of the invasion and details of German military plans. Stalin not only refused to believe any of it but also kept sending shipments of Russian food and war materials to Germany, although Hitler was no longer sending anything in return.

Stalin defended his delusions with his customary ferocity. The Soviet press threatened anyone who even discussed the possibility of danger from Germany. But underneath Stalin was gripped by a paralyzing depression that was marked by indecisiveness, pessimism, and anxiety. Throughout the spring of 1941, he oscillated between worry about leaving his country defenseless and fear of doing anything to provoke Hitler. On June 13, Stalin turned down a general's request to put certain border areas on war alert. Two days later, he turned around and sent additional rifle divisions to the threatened regions —but insisted nevertheless that the border districts not prepare for war.

When the invasion actually began on June 22, Stalin refused to believe that it was anything but, said Khrushchev, "a provocation on the part of the German field commander acting independently of Hitler. Stalin was so afraid of war that even when the Germans tried to take us by surprise and wipe out our resistance, Stalin convinced himself that Hitler would keep his word and wouldn't really attack us."

Stalin clung tenaciously to his deluded version of reality even when it was clear German tanks were rolling across the border. He refused to permit Russian soldiers to fire back, or his generals to make any decisions for hours.

STALIN COLLAPSES

The belated realization that the Germans were, in fact, attacking threw the Soviet dictator into a severely disabling depression. When General Georgy Zhukov telephoned his first report, Stalin was unable to say a word in reply. He held a meeting of the Politburo and again remained silent, unable to tell his nation that it was at war, Foreign Minister Vyacheslav Molotov having to make the broadcast for him. Depression gave way briefly to rage when Stalin learned that the Red Army was fleeing from the German Panzers. He coped with the crisis by taking refuge in fantasy, issuing unfulfillable orders for Soviet forces to go on the offensive and annihilate the enemy.

Then Stalin retreated to his dacha at Kuntsevo where, according to Khrushchev, he spent the next several days in seclusion, drinking. The dictator's daughter noted that he was confused during this period and uncharacteristically kind. On hearing that the Germans were advancing at a rate of 20 miles per day, Stalin replied despairingly to secret police chief Lavrenti Beria, "Everything is lost. I give up. Lenin left us a proletarian state, and now we've been caught with our pants down and let the whole thing go to shit."

Stalin remained in isolation for a week, refusing to give orders or take part in consultations, refusing to see or speak to anyone. When, on June 2, he heard that the Germans had surrounded main elements of his defensive force, he panicked and, overwhelmed by the pessimism of his depression, felt certain that the war was already lost. Lack of directives from Stalin compounded the problems of the Soviet forces, allowing divisions and entire armies to be surrounded and destroyed within days of the start of the invasion. Historian Roy Medvedev states that "Stalin's absence from his post as head of state and the party from June 23 to the beginning of July was an important reason why the Nazis penetrated so swiftly and so deeply into the USSR." Stalin's only contribution to his nation's defense that June was to order the arrest and execution of a number of his defeated generals and their subordinates. He also ordered the shooting of "rumor-mongers, panic-spreaders, and cowards," dealing with his own defects in his habitual manner.

RAGE AND PANIC

Stalin returned to the exercise of his responsibilities only when members of the Politburo visited him and insisted that he respond to the national emergency. Stalin's resumption of activity did not improve matters, however. Setbacks intensified his depression, which made him panicky and indecisive, while his orders interfered with what his generals were trying to do, often generating frightful consequences. Nikolai Voronov, Deputy Commissar of Defense, described his leader as "depressed, nervous, and off-balance. When he gave assignments, he demanded that they be completed in unbelievably short times without considering real possibilities."

It was not until eleven days after the Germans invaded Russia that Stalin could bring himself to address his nation. He "spoke in a sort of hollow, colorless voice, halting and breathing heavily," recalled a Soviet citizen remembering the broadcast's disturbing effect. "Stalin seemed ill, seemed to be speaking with an effort. This was no way to raise his listeners' morale and enthusiasm."

The dictator's depression soon took on an irritable coloring. He went into a wild rage on July 17 when Smolensk was captured. Twelve days later, General Zhukov asked permission to retreat again and Stalin, refusing, replaced him. In August, Stalin's sister-in-law, Yevgenia Alliluyeva, visited him. He imprisoned her later, perhaps for what she saw then. She relates, "I had never seen Joseph so crushed and in such confusion. I came to him, thinking I would find support, hoping to get some encouragement. Novgorod, the city of my birth, had just been surrendered to the Germans and I was in a panic. I was even more frightened when I found he was almost in a state of panic himself! He said, 'Things are very bad, very bad! Get yourself evacuated. I can't stay in Moscow.' I left completely lost; I thought this was the end." Summing up his leader's depression and demoralization, Khrushchev later attested that "Stalin lost control and even lost his will during the period of our retreat from the Germans."

DEFEAT IN DEPTH

When Stalin finally recovered sufficiently to resume his responsibilities, his orders were still based on denial of painful realities and on paranoid suspicions of his generals. When in September, Kiev, the capital of the Ukraine, was about to be surrounded, Stalin once more denied permission to evacuate and replaced the Kiev commander. When a general of higher rank made the same request, Stalin called him a panic monger. By the time the dictator faced reality and gave permission for retreat, it was too late. The Germans took about 700,000 prisoners.

As the world watched, the German Wehrmacht swept into Russia, capturing in only four weeks an area double the size of France. Although many concluded that the Russians were poor soldiers, the Germans' initial success was actually due in large measure to Stalin's mental illness. Prompted by paranoia, he had gutted the Soviet military command and the leadership of the defense industry. Manic overconfidence made him refuse to prepare for defensive warfare. Depression made him deny the imminence of invasion, the invasion itself, and the desperate straits of his forces as the Wehrmacht rolled across Russia. Depression put him completely out of commission during the crucial first week of the war, and his irrational military leadership afterward was an ongoing catastrophe.

Stalin's murderous tyranny inspired his fellow citizens, for the first time in Russian history, to join an invader: by the time the war ended, a million Soviet officers and soldiers had chosen to fight on the side of the Germans.

THE MAGIC WARRIOR

Stalin's disabling depressions lasted well into the fall of 1941 and intensified when the German forces began their climactic thrust toward Moscow. General P. Zelov observed a severely depressed Stalin during a discussion of the defense of the city. "In eight years he had aged twenty. His eyes lacked their former firmness, and confidence was no longer sensed in his voice." Stalin ordered the evacuation of women and children from Moscow on October 12. Four days later he fled himself, leaving the city without government. The militia and NKVD also disappeared and panic prevailed.

Stalin rallied more quickly this time and returned to the city three days later, declaring that Moscow would be held at all costs. And it was—partly through the excellent leadership of Zhukov and partly because the German tanks and men became hopelessly bogged down in the autumn mud and then were frozen in place by the Russian winter.

Until the turning point came, Stalin remained extremely agitated and gloomy. But with Moscow now safe, and Zhukov staging effective counter-attacks, Stalin's manic assertiveness returned. "I found myself confronted with a new man," Khrushchev recalled. "He had pulled himself together, straightened up, and was acting like a real soldier. He'd also begun to think of himself as a great military strategist, which made it harder than ever to argue with him."

Stalin's new confidence was a mixed blessing. Now he entertained manic delusions that all was possible and that the German forces were no longer superior in numbers and equipment. His manic optimism made him insist that Soviet troops attack everywhere despite the horrendous losses they had endured, and he refused General Zhukov's request for time to allow the army to rest and reorganize. The result was that Russian casualties continued to surpass those of the enemy. This further weakened the Red Army and opened the way for the German victories that would come in the summer of 1942.

The dictator insisted that the next major German offensive would again be against Moscow—despite warnings from his intelligence that Hitler was planning to attack southward toward the oilfields of Baku and the Trans-Caucasus. Disregarding all evidence, Stalin remained convinced of his infallibility and again his delusions brought disaster. The Germans turned away from Moscow and overran huge areas in Southern Russia, destroying Soviet armies in the process.

Stalin's manic depression made him quite unfit to make military decisions, yet his manic ego insisted on controlling his generals as though they were puppets. His paranoia inspired him to make frequent changes of commanders, further disorganizing his forces, and he gave the greatest responsibilities to those who were incompetent but docile. His fear of the prestige of capable generals was greater than his desire for victories. Stalin also undermined his relationships with his generals. He would curse them and hang up the phone when he did not want to give them reinforcements, or when they protested his movement of their armies. He vented his fury on them when his decisions produced disasters, although the generals had only followed his orders. Depression occasionally caused severe problems, too. Essential supplies had to be left behind and even entire armies lost when Stalin was not in the mood to come to the telephone to give the necessary commands. Occasionally he gave military orders when drunk.

GENERALISSIMO EGO

Stalin's most consistent and grievous fault as a military leader, however, was his conviction of infallibility coupled with his manic drive to protect his ego. Anything smacking of defeat was therefore insupportable. On one occasion he even refused to sign his own order to scuttle the warships in Leningrad harbor—ships that shortly thereafter were seized by the Germans. It was this self-regard that also forbade the surrender of any ground to the enemy. Like Hitler's, Stalin's ego rejected the very notion of retreat. Stalin's attitude toward strategic withdrawal was expressed in an order that could have been one of Hitler's: "If so much as a single soldier retreats a single meter . . ., the following will be shot: the commander of the front, the members of the military council, the commanders of the armies, and the chiefs of the political units." Medvedev notes: "He was short-sighted and cruel, careless of losses, unwilling and unable to fight with little loss of blood, little interested in the fate of the common people." Stalin did not care how many died to spare him humiliation.

Stalin's ego could not tolerate any disagreement with his plans. Naturally, this aroused secret rebellion in some military leaders. One Soviet marshal admitted in 1968, "That half-educated priest just interfered with everything. We had to deceive him, whatever absurd order he gave, we said 'Yessir!' then went on our own."

Stalin gave his officers other reasons for deceiving him. His reaction to bad news was often to order the arrest and punishment as traitors of the military leaders involved. Those who merely reported bad news risked arrest for spreading panic. As always, this kind of irrationality resulted in the withholding of any information that could set off a dangerous reaction, so the tyrant's fantastic version of reality was left undisturbed. Communication between Stalin and his generals became full of static, as the paranoid dictator was afraid to share information with anyone and told his generals as little as possible. With all the problems Stalin's manic depression created, it seems miraculous that he and his generals ever managed to cooperate sufficiently to win the war. Part of the explanation is that Hitler and his military men had almost identical problems. Both Hitler's and Stalin's generals were more fearful of their leader than they were of the enemy, while the dictators lived in constant terror of being overthrown by their own generals.

PRISONERS OF PARANOIA

Not even the great conflict could deflect Stalin's paranoia from his fellow citizens. After 1942 all Soviet residents were subject to arrest for making suspicious remarks, that is, saying anything that was negative about the USSR or favorable to another country. Even inmates of prison camps could be arrested for this "crime" and subjected to additional punishment.

Nor were the defenders of the nation spared. Thirteen months after the invasion, military officers arrested during the purge of 1936–1938 were still being executed. Secret police continued to spy on all ranks of the military throughout the war and maintained a network of informers among members of the armed forces. All military personnel accused of disobedience or cowardice were either shot or sent to special prisoner battalions. These were often used as human shields, forced to advance into enemy fire in front of regular troops. The secret police maintained blocking battalions that followed regular troops in order to shoot anyone who retreated. It was a crime to surrender and even relatives of those taken prisoner were arrested. The secret police executed entire army units that had been cut off from their own forces even after they had heroically fought their way back. Because Stalin saw anyone who was captured as a traitor, he dealt those unfortunates another vengeful blow, refusing to permit the International Red Cross to offer them any assistance while they suffered and died in Hitler's gruesome prisoner of war camps.

VICTORIES AND DEATH TRIPS

Stalin's manic high mood lasted from the winter of 1941 into the summer of 1942, and was evident when he played the amiable host to Churchill in the Kremlin in August. His mood was reinforced the following winter with the annihilation of a quarter-milllion-man German army at Stalingrad. He celebrated by making himself a generalissimo, a marshal, and by bestowing upon himself two medals set in diamonds.

By May of 1943, however, Stalin's euphoria had worn off. He was slipping into an anxious depression, unable to decide whether or not to launch a summer offensive; he was also fearful of the German offensive that was apparently imminent. By July, though, there was much encouraging news: The German defeat in Africa was followed by the Anglo-American landing in Sicily. The Red Army was pushing the Germans steadily westward. By December, when Stalin met with Churchill and Roosevelt at Teheran, the Soviet dictator was in a confident mood again. That New Year's Eve he felt merry enough to throw an impromptu party for his generals.

Nineteen forty-four was another year in which Stalin's moods were predominantly manic. At one supper that he gave, Stalin announced enthusiastically: "The war will soon be over. We shall recover in fifteen or twenty years and then we will have another go at it!" The Allied landing in Normandy in June so pleased the dictator that he allowed Soviet newspapers to list some of the military supplies that the United States, England, and Canada had been sending since 1941. His mood was so benign that he permitted American and

British periodicals to circulate in the USSR and allowed foreign films to be shown. Censorship was loosened; some of the victims of the purge were declared innocent. Soviet citizens began to hope that peace would bring a relaxation of Stalin's oppressive rule. The Soviet government also proclaimed that countries being occupied by the Red Army would not be required to become Communist—another unkept promise.

The Yugoslav writer Milovan Djilas saw Stalin at a banquet the Soviet dictator gave during the winter of 1944–1945. Stalin behaved like a textbook manic depressive, his moods fluctuating extraordinarily over a period of only a few hours. According to Djilas, "He spoke agitatedly about the sufferings of the Red Army and about the horrors that it was forced to undergo. . . . He wept." But then an extreme change of mood took place. "He proposed frequent toasts," Djilas recalled, "flattered one person, joked with another, needled a third, kissed my wife because she was a Serb, and again shed tears over the hardships of the Red Army and Yugoslav ingratitude."

THE JOYS OF PEACE

Even in victory Stalin's vengefulness and paranoia continued unabated. As the Germans withdrew from Russian territory, he began to take revenge on those Soviet citizens who had sided with or given any help to the enemy. He also indiscriminately punished loyal citizens who shared the nationality of the disloyal. In 1943 and 1944, Stalin uprooted entire Soviet nationalities, totaling some four or five million people, from their homes. As usual, his victims were herded onto freight cars without extra clothing or other belongings and without food, water, or heat. When the cars were unlocked at their destinations in Siberia, Ovseyenko relates, "the corpses of the children were carried out first, then those of the adults." Those who resisted shipment from their villages were locked in sheds and cremated alive.

Paranoia did not permit Stalin to distinguish between being captured by the enemy and trying to escape from Soviet control. Therefore most of the Soviet citizens who had been put in Nazi concentration camps, and the millions of Soviet soldiers who had been prisoners of war, were condemend for "high treason." When they reached the USSR, they were sent directly to Stalin's camps without being allowed to see their families.

The dictator's paranoid xenophobia had an additional deadly fallout. Anyone living in an area that the Germans had occupied was examined for political reliability by the secret police. Many were "reindoctrinated," that is, freighted to a camp or killed outright. Stalin's fears of the dangers of foreign contact were so great that soldiers who had fought their way into Germany and the Balkans were not allowed at demobilization to return to their own homes, but had to work far away, among strangers, to reduce the likelihood of their talking about life in the West.

THE BODY COUNT

Hitler's war was, of course, an immense disaster for the Russian people, but it was made worse at virtually every turn by Stalin's tyranny and irrationality. First he refused to allow his own country to take proper defensive measures. Then his disregard of warnings of the oncoming German invasion and dereliction of duty after the invasion helped Hitler's armies capture three and a half million Soviet soldiers during the first three months of the war. His refusal to permit retreats at Kiev and Smolensk cost a million casualties and another two million captured. His Crimean offensive cost the Red Army 200,000 casualties in a single month; 300,000 more men were lost in Stalin's attempt to retake Kharkov. Medvedev states, "With other leadership the army could have defeated the Nazi aggressor . . . much farther west and much sooner. Hundreds of towns and tens of thousands of villages would not have been destroyed."

Soviet demographers have calculated that more than 27 million Soviet citizens lost their lives in World War II. Millions more were left crippled. Some 25 million were reduced to living in caves, mud huts, and dugouts. Most of European Russia's agriculture, industry, cities, and towns were destroyed. Much of this loss was the consequence of Stalin's paranoia and grandiose manic depressive delusions.

The only saving grace was that Stalin faced another dictator equally handicapped as a military leader by his own manic depression. Often grandiosely overconfident, both tyrants needlessly sacrificed lives while attempting the impossible. In times of crisis they denied reality and were thus unable to respond effectively. Their colossal egos would not permit their forces to retreat, regardless of the cost. Their paranoia and insistence on total control severely reduced the effectiveness of their professional military men. Each of them served the enemy magnificently.

12

A Fearful Triumph

A PAINFUL PEACE

Stalin was the most successful dictator of modern times if power alone is the criterion. During his final years he ruled an empire more vast, more populous, than that of Hitler, his nearest competitor, and he was General Secretary nineteen years longer than Hitler was Chancellor. As for Stalin's Russian predecessors, he controlled a greater part of his subjects' lives than any of the tsars. No law, no organ of the government or the military, no institution of any kind, could withstand his will. He was supreme ruler of the largest country in the world, and could have spent the post-war period enjoying his achievements. But paranoid manic depressives rarely end their lives in tranquil satisfaction, and Stalin was pursued through his last years by the same fears, rages, and depressions he had always known. "Even beyond the borders of Russia there were those who burned incense at his feet," his daughter, Svetlana, observed. "He should have been happy, he should have lived and enjoyed a full life, he should have loved everyone around him. But he could not; he was incapable of rejoicing over the harvest he had reaped."

During his remaining years, Stalin became increasingly more reclusive. His paranoia again rose to the point of inspiring a purge almost equal to that of the 1930s. So long as Stalin lived under his delusions, he could not let his people live in peace.

Drought came to the Ukraine in 1946, creating a desperate situation for an area that had been devastated by the war and that lacked everything. Casualties had severely reduced manpower; housing, equipment of every kind, and storage facilities had been destroyed. However, the Ukraine had been the grainery of the Soviet Union before the war and Stalin demanded that it produce again, quickly. Khrushchev recorded that the quota for grain "had been calculated not on the basis of how much we really could produce, but on the basis of how much the State thought it could beat out of us." Stalin's quotas had to be met regardless of whether there remained anything with which to feed the Ukrainians. In the ensuing famine some of the starving resorted to cannibalism, as had happened in the 1930s.

During the famine of 1931–1932 doctors had been forbidden to register starvation as a cause of death. Stalin's response to this second famine that his policies caused was the same: denial. Khrushchev sent him a detailed report of conditions in the Ukraine and requested that some grain be left to feed the people, with the issuance of ration cards to assure fair distribution. "In reply," he reports, "Stalin sent me the rudest, insulting telegram. I was a dubious character, he said." When Khrushchev visited Moscow to tell him about the famine, Stalin screamed, "You're being soft-bellied! They're deceiving you! They're counting on being able to appeal to your sentimentality when they report things like that. They're trying to force you to give them all your reserves." As he did when his excessively rapid collectivization caused the famine of the 1930s, Stalin insisted that this famine was a fiction and he refused to relieve it in any way. In his perfect USSR, famine could not exist. He remained incapable of coping with, or even admitting the existence of, serious problems that threatened his ego.

PARANOIA AND PERSECUTION

A heart ailment kept Stalin inactive for several weeks during the winter of 1946–1947. When he recovered, his temper and paranoia took a permanent turn for the worse. Khrushchev noted: "Stalin became even more capricious, irritable, and brutal; in particular his suspicion grew. His persecution mania reached unbelievable dimensions."

Milovan Djilas noted the change in 1948, at one of Stalin's dinners. Missing was the camaraderie of earlier years. The dictator had become, Djilas observed, "stubborn, sharp, suspicious whenever anyone disagreed with him. He even cut Molotov, and I could feel the tension between them."

In the same year, Svetlana observed paranoia invading her father's private relationships. "He was embittered against the entire world and no longer believed anyone. 'You, too, make anti-Soviet statements,' he said to me at the time, quite seriously. It had become impossible to talk to him. I avoided him and he had no particular wish to see me."

Paranoia prompted Stalin to further persecutions as soon as new populations came within his reach. In 1945–1946 he uprooted more than three million citizens of German origin from Czechoslovakia. Hundreds committed suicide rather than be taken; thousands were killed in the process of being rounded up, and the survivors were sent to camps in the Soviet Union.

The Yalta agreement allowed the Soviets to seize two million "displaced persons," including Russians who had been living in Europe since the Russian Revolution. These, too, were freighted to Soviet camps. From 1945 to 1950, one out of every six Moldavians was exiled, sent to camps, or executed as Stalin continued his vengenace against Soviet nationalities.

In 1946, the dictator inaugurated a fanatical purging of everything Western or slightly liberal from Soviet life. The arts and artists became special targets, composers Sergei Prokofiev and Dmitri Shostakovich being told to "purify" their work. Soviet citizens risked arrest if they answered any questions asked by foreigners. The USSR became again a vast jail for its citizens. Foreigners who married Russians could not take their families with them if they left the country.

Both xenophobia and paranoia contributed to Stalin's refusal of Marshall Plan aid, though the condition of his war-ravaged country should have made him eager to accept any relief that was offered. Stalin also insisted that Poland and Czechoslovakia refuse American assistance.

MINI-PURGES

The old paranoid fear of possible rivals also continued. Andrei Zhdanov, who had apparently been chosen by Stalin as his successor, fell from favor in 1948 and was poisoned, although his death was attributed to a "heart attack." As usual, when he eliminated someone possessing power, Stalin purged anyone who had been close to the victim. Since Zhdanov's base was Leningrad, the entire local leadership of the party (including the members of the city government), many of Leningrad's leading citizens, and thousands of other inhabitants were arrested or simply disappeared. Party members in Moscow who owed their advancements to Zhdanov were also caught in Stalin's net. The Georgian developed the delusion that all these people were conspiring to make Leningrad the capital of the USSR.

The ritual of humiliation and vengeance was enacted again as it had been in 1936–1938: torture, false confessions, and public "trials." Khrushchev attested that the accused "had already been sentenced a considerable time before the sentence was officially passed, and even before the trial began. In fact, they had been sentenced by Stalin himself at the time of their arrest." Stalin's vengeance extended to Leningrad itself. The museum commemorating the city's heroic 900-day resistance to the German seige was eliminated and its director exiled to Siberia.

Stalin's anti-Semitism, another expression of his paranoia, became conspicuous in 1948. In May of that year, the USSR recognized the new State of

Israel, Stalin's motive being that he wanted to weaken the British Empire. However, when Israeli Prime Minister Golda Meir's visit to Moscow was greeted by thousands of Jews cheering in the city streets, Stalin read the demonstration as a sign that Soviet Jews favored Israel over Russia. From then on, Israel was denounced and Soviet foreign policy became pro-Arab. Soviet Jews were deprived of their rights to publish periodicals, newspapers, and books in Yiddish; to maintain a Yiddish theater; and to have Yiddish taught their children in the state schools. Through stringent quotas Jews were denied higher education and many sorts of employment. Jewish artists, writers, and scientists were arrested and imprisoned, deported, or shot. Jews were dismissed from positions in the party and the government, from posts in universities and scientific institutes. They were even fired from factories.

THE PUPPET-MAKER

The rising paranoia of Stalin's post-war years led him, in 1947, to reverse his previous position allowing the satellite nations to develop communism according to their own circumstances and requirements. He henceforth insisted that the Soviet pattern be followed without any deviation. His attempts to increase his control over these countries are indications of Stalin's growing feeling of insecurity. Fear prompted him to create a barricade of subservient nations around the USSR.

Stalin had begun the necessary maneuvers as early as 1943, pushing his armies to race across Eastern Europe to Berlin in order to establish his control before the British and Americans could challenge it. Grandiosity also contributed to his lust for territory, which he acquired in Asia as well. As for the spread of communism per se, Stalin had no interest in it unless the Communists promoting revolution were his puppets.

Stalin was interested only in his own power and security, not in ideology. He had a consistent history of hostility to foreign Communist movements. In 1935 he tried to woo Hitler by offering him a free hand to destroy the German Communists. The offer was not accepted, but Stalin weakened the German Communists on his own, by forbidding them to join the left-wing groups in resisting the rise of Hitler. At that time, his fear that the Communists and socialists would jointly turn against him was greater than his fear of Nazism. He responded tardily to the Spanish Communists' requests for aid during their civil war and insisted on receiving the gold reserves of Spain as payment. During World War II, Stalin refused aid to an uprising of Slovakian Communists against the Germans, and neglected the Yugoslavs as well. For years, Tito was helped only by the British. The Yugoslav leader finally cabled Stalin: "If you cannot send us assistance, then at least do not hamper us."

The Soviet dictator did nothing for the Communists of Greece, France, or Italy after the war, and his aid to China was niggardly. He had tried to discourage Mao Tse-tung over the years, hoping that Mao, the Japanese, and the right-wing Chinese would annihilate each other, leaving the Stalinist Communists to inherit China. "He helped revolutions only up to a certain point— up to where he could control them," Djilas observed, "but he was ready to leave them in the lurch when they slipped out of his grasp."

After the war, Stalin tried to gain perfect and detailed control over all of the Communist parties in the world, often to their detriment. Khrushchev said: "You see to what Stalin's mania for greatness led. He completely lost consciousness of reality; he demonstrated his suspicions and haughtiness not only in relation to individuals in the USSR, but in relations to whole parties and nations." Stalin's paranoid suspicions and fear of foreigners took bizarre, almost comic, forms. During a visit to Moscow, North Vietnamese leader Ho Chi Minh asked Stalin to autograph a magazine. "Stalin gave Ho his autograph," Khrushchev reported, "but shortly afterwards had the magazine stolen back from him because he was worried about how Ho might use it."

Among Stalin's first acts in the satellite countries after his armies had overrun them was to strip them of agricultural and industrial goods that had survived the war, including entire factories and, in some cases, whole industries. Thereafter he made them subsidize the Soviet Union by selling their goods below market prices to their giant neighbor, which the USSR sold on the world market for a large profit. In return, the satellites had to buy Soviet goods at whatever price was asked.

Having turned his back on the Marshall Plan, Stalin established his own version, Comecon. This, however, was a Marshall Plan in reverse. Instead of the larger country aiding the smaller ones, Russia offered no aid to the satellites, but merely continued to squeeze them. Thus Stalin achieved two goals at once: enriching the Soviet Union while simultaneously weakening its neighbors.

In addition to serving as shields and economic resources for the Soviet Union, the satellites were useful to Stalin as tools. Roy Medvedev notes that "he regarded the leaders of the new socialist countries as his vassals, obliged to obey him without demur in foreign and internal policy." Stalin guaranteed his domination of the satellites by selecting the native-born leaders for each country, by subordinating the local armed forces to Soviet control, and by directing the local secret police from the Kremlin. Furthermore, satellite countries were not permitted to initiate any relationships with each other: there must be no opportunity for them to combine against Stalin.

DAVID AND GOLIATH

The one satellite leader who successfully defied Stalin was Yugoslavia's Josip Broz Tito. Already suspect because he did not owe his rise to Stalin, Tito also committed the cardinal sin of attempting to assist another Iron Curtain country, Albania, without Stalin's permission. On March 27, 1948, Stalin wrote Tito criticizing his actions and threatening him with assassination. "I will shake my little finger," Stalin announced to Khrushchev, "and there will be no more Tito." But Tito did not fall—or back off. Stalin "did everything possible to provoke a fight," Tito recorded, "and he had his forces massed on our frontiers in case an opportunity should arise." None did. When Stalin ordered Tito's assassination, the Yugoslav leader sent a letter back that said, "Stalin, you've sent seven men after me—with pistols, grenades, and poison. If I send one, I won't have to send another."

Unable to destroy Tito, Stalin turned on the leadership of most of the other satellite countries: Albania, Bulgaria, Czechoslovakia, Hungary, Poland, and Romania. He instituted purges reminiscent of the 1930s, complete with torture, false confessions to absurd accusations, and "show trials" from 1948 through 1952. Many of the satellites' leaders were brought to the USSR to be dealt with there, while Soviet labor camps were filled with fresh victims from the satellite nations.

As did the Great Purge of the 1930s, the satellite purges served several purposes. Communist leaders with their own national followings were replaced by Stalin's choices, men entirely dependent on his support. Complaints against the fallen standard of living resulting from accelerated collectivization and industrialization were silenced, and the satellites became, to a large degree, terrorized police states with their own prison camp populations. Furthermore, the purges diminished the likelihood of another Tito emerging on the borders of the Soviet Union.

THE AGING GOD

The realization that he was growing old caused the paranoid dictator added anxiety. The approaching end to his rule increased his vulnerability. Signs of age were unmistakable: "Every year it became more and more obvious that Stalin was weakening mentally as well as physically," Khrushchev noted.

This was particularly evident from his eclipses of mind and losses of memory. When he was well and sober, he was still a formidable leader, but he was declining fast. I recall once he turned to Bulganin and started to say something but couldn't remember his name. Stalin looked at him intently and said "You there, what's your name?" "Bulganin." "Of course, Bulganin! That's what I was going to say." Stalin became very unnerved when this kind of thing happened. He didn't want others to notice. But these slips of memory occurred more and more frequently, and they used to drive him crazy.

As usual, when some occurrence or condition threatened Stalin's ego, his response was to project the fault onto others. He became angry at his elderly servants because *they* were showing signs of age.

The passing years, however, failed to diminish Stalin's aggressiveness. In March 1948, he closed Berlin to the West and did not lift his blockade until the summer of 1949, when the success of the American airlift had proven his blockade futile. In the winter of 1949–1950, he ordered the head of the Japanese Communist party, Sanzo Nosaga, to seize Japan by force. Nosaga refused, explaining that it was not possible with American occupation forces still in place. In 1950, Stalin encouraged the North Koreans to invade South Korea. Even when a large-scale war resulted, Stalin discouraged the North Koreans from negotiating for peace, hoping the warring forces would destroy each other so that he could acquire the entire Korean peninsula.

Mania was the mood of the summer of 1950. Stalin gandiosely presented himself as an expert on linguistics and began publishing articles on the subject. He also released his "Great Stalinist Plan for Remaking Nature," which called for using atomic bombs to rearrange the geography of the Soviet Union so as to improve its climate and agricultural productivity. A 700-mile canal in Central Asia was one of many impractical projects abandoned after Stalin died. Meanwhile, nothing was done about the ruins and slums that the war had left behind.

In the winter of 1951, the fever of Stalin's paranoia began to rise again. He accused groups in Georgia of plotting, with Western assistance, to make the Republic of Georgia a part of Turkey. Khrushchev observed: "Could the Georgians, comparing the situation in their republic with the hard situation of the working masses in Turkey, be aspiring to join Turkey? . . . . As it developed, there was no nationalistic organization in Georgia." Laboring under another paranoid delusion, Stalin also accused Soviet Jews of conspiring to establish a new Jewish State—a second Israel, as it were—in the Crimean part of the USSR.

By 1952 Stalin had developed his own plans for creating a Jewish ghetto in the Soviet Union. His idea: to deport all Soviet Jews to Birobidzhan, in Central Asia. He told the Politburo: "There is danger of a pogrom against the Jews. Many cases of hoodlum attacks on prominent Jews have been reported. I think, comrades, we must save and protect our Jews. The best thing would be to relocate them." The few who were permitted to remain, he said, would wear yellow stars on their sleeves. His kind intentions drew vigorous protests from Politburo members who reminded him that they had not fought Hitler in order to imitate him. Stalin became furious and shortly broke diplomatic relations with Israel. Only his death prevented a Nazi-style persecution of Soviet Jews.

The "Doctors' Plot," which involved six Jewish and three non-Jewish medical specialists, was announced on January 13, 1953. Stalin maintained that the most eminent physicians in the USSR were British and American spies who had, over the previous eight years, killed three marshals, a general, an admiral, a secretary of the Central Committee, and Andrei Zhdanov—whose death Stalin himself had ordered. *Pravda* called the physicians "vile spies" and "murderers in the guise of professors." When a skeptical party member wrote to Stalin suggesting that further investigations be made, he was confined to a psychiatric hospital for two years.

Torture extracted the usual false confessions. As he gave copies of the confessions to members of the Politburo, Stalin said, "You are blind like young kittens. What will happen without me? The country will perish because you do not know how to recognize enemies." Thereafter he refused to allow any doctors near him and insisted on medicating himself. After his death the doctors were exonerated and those still alive were released.

A DUBIOUS DEMISE

Signs that still another purge was in the making appeared in 1952. Longtime foreign minister Molotov was among the first to be targeted. Khrushchev's memoirs describe how Stalin selected his victim:

> [I]t suddenly came into Stalin's head that Molotov was an agent of American imperialism. And what was the evidence for this charge? It seems that when Molotov was in the United States he traveled from Washington to New York by train. Stalin reasoned that if Molotov traveled by train, then he must have had his own private railway car. And if he had his own private railway car, then where did he get the money? Hence, Molotov must have sold himself to the Americans.

An investigation cleared Molotov, but Stalin's belief in his guilt remained unchanged. He sent Molotov's wife to prison, treated his longtime colleague as a pariah, and, Khrushchev believed, would have done away with Molotov had his own death not intervened.

Stalin also denounced a number of other Politburo members to the Central Committee, including Beria, the former head of the secret police. Stalin also enlarged the Politburo so as to have their successors in place. "He's going to wipe us all out," Beria said shortly before Stalin's death. Panic hit the Politburo as members surrounded themselves with guards or went into hiding.

This old guard was saved when, suddenly and rather mysteriously, Stalin's political power and his health both began to fail. On February 17, 1953, *Izvestia* announced the sudden death of the chief of Kremlin Security. There were suspicions that he had been killed. Stalin seemed to have lost his grip on the military when the Red Army Chief of Staff was replaced five days later by someone of whom the dictator disapproved. The next day, February 22, all Soviet media abruptly stopped a pre-purge vigilance campaign, and the witch-hunt associated with the "Doctors' Plot" terminated. Three days later, on February 25, the arrests of Jews were abruptly discontinued. Stalin's personal bodyguard disappeared.

Khrushchev claimed that Stalin was in good health and boisterous spirits at a late-night party on February 28, which was also attended by the dictator's prospective Politburo victims. Supposedly, Stalin did not become ill until March 1, and was not known to be ill until 3:00 A.M. of March 2, when he was found at his dacha, lying unconscious on the floor.

According to Khrushchev, Stalin remained unconscious for most of the next three days, paralyzed on the right side and unable to speak. Svetlana, summoned belatedly to her father's side, said, "He literally choked to death as we watched." The autopsy stated that a hemorrhage in the left cerebral hemisphere had killed Stalin at 9:50 P.M. on March 5.

It was rumored, however, that Beria had poisoned the dictator, and it seems likely, in view of subsequent events, that something of this sort did occur. Within hours of Stalin's death, Beria had not only reasserted control over the secret police, but had also arrested the commandants of the Moscow Military District, the Moscow city garrison, and the Kremlin guards. Large numbers of Beria's troops patrolled all the key points in Moscow, which was surrounded with NKVD tanks and flame throwers. Trains were not permitted to enter the city. The next day, what amounted to a *coup d'état* took place, with Georgi Malenkov—who had fallen out of Stalin's favor—being swiftly named Prime Minister. That Stalin's death itself was suspicious would seem to be indicated by the fact that within weeks, three of the nine doctors who had signed the autopsy report on Stalin's corpse had vanished.

Khrushchev later claimed that "right up to his very death, Stalin could express himself clearly and concisely." Why, then, were Stalin's policies terminated and the men he relied on removed while he was supposedly in good health and sound mind? This puzzle can have only one solution: Khrushchev was lying. The government was taken over before Stalin's death, but while he was helpless, by the same men who later assumed the leadership of the Soviet Union. Apparently, there was a conspiracy among those whom Stalin was about to destroy. No one except these people is known to have been with him between February 17 and the morning of March 2 when Stalin could no longer speak. The speed and coordination with which Beria's army of secret police occupied Moscow, as well as the ease with which Stalin's prospective victims took power and eliminated their opposition, suggest that careful and elaborate preparations were made prior to the dictator's convenient demise.

STALIN'S LEGACY

Although many Soviet citizens felt a great sense of loss when Stalin died, they had little reason to do so. He left the nation's agriculture in worse condition than it had been during the tenure of the last tsar. Stalin is credited with having advanced the industrialization of the USSR, but this would have taken place under anyone, and was well begun before the Russian Revolution. It surely would have gone farther without the tyrant's mass persecutions. Roy Medvedev poses the question: "Would not solidarity between the people and the government have been stronger had there been no mass repression? . . . Would not economic and cultural progress have been much greater if Stalin had not destroyed thousands upon thousands of scientists, engineers, teachers, doctors, writers?" Medvedev's conclusion: "Stalin was for thirty years the helmsman of the ship of state, clutching its steering wheel in a grip of death. Dozens of times he steered it onto reefs and shoals and far off course. Should we be grateful to him because he did not manage to sink it altogether?"

For the privilege of being ruled by a grandiose, paranoid, manic depressive head of state for more than three decades, the people of the Soviet Union paid with perhaps forty million lives. During World War II, Stalin's delusions added millions more to the already horrendous death count. Yet even that does not express the extent of the calamity Stalin visited on his country. Part of the tragedy of the Soviet Union was that Stalin's irrationality and his delusions continued to darken his nation after his death, feeding its paranoia, xenophobia, hatreds, and prejudices.

Part Four

Three Sick Men

13

Napoleon's Lunacy and Success

The previous chapters have shown the effects of manic depression on the political and military decisions made by Napoleon, Hitler, and Stalin. In the remaining two parts of our study, we shall talk more about the personalities of each dictator as their illness shaped them—giving them uncommon advantages in some instances and severely handicapping them in others. As no two personalities are exactly alike, so no two human beings experience manic depression in precisely the same way. Part Four will show the extent to which Napoleon, Hitler, and Stalin differed. Part Five will discuss their likenesses: those extreme and most distorting symptoms of manic depression that they shared, the symptoms that turned them into tyrants.

Manic depression is the only emotional disorder that can transport someone to both high office and certifiable insanity. Had depression alone dominated Napoleon's life, he would not have become the emperor of France and the most dangerous man of his time. Depression would have deprived him of ambition—and of any hope of playing a role on the stage of history. But he was not simply a depressive, and it was the manic enhancement of his undeniable talent and intelligence that enabled him to take advantage of the opportunities provided by his time and place to become the unprecedented phenomenon that was Napoleon I. Mania was the secret of Napoleon's success.

MANIC BONUSES

When Napoleon was manic he could be playful, funny, and charming. In such moods he was agreeable to everyone, including servants. One of them recalled that "nothing could equal the gentle gaiety and charm of his conversation. . . . Endowed with a lively wit, a superior intelligence, and extraordinary tact, he surprised and enchanted people the most in his moments of abandon and chatting." Bonaparte's charm was a considerable political asset.

The currently fashionable word "charisma" also applies to Napoleon, to his amazing compound of enthusiasm, ambition, and self-confidence coupled with a drive to dominate any situation or person, a gift for acting or at least for self-dramatization, and boundless sexual energy. All of these are also elements of mania. Every leader needs supporters who will execute his will, look after his interests, and promote his projects as they do their own. Even when he was in captivity, Napoleon retained his charismatic ability to dominate. Count Balmain, the Russian commissioner on St. Helena, wrote:

> The most astonishing thing of all is the influence which this man—a captive, deprived of a throne—wields on anyone who comes near him. . . . The French tremble at the sight of him. . . . The English approach him only with something like awe. Even those who stand guard over him jealously seek his glances, and are avid for one little word from him. No one dares to approach him on a basis of equality.

Augment charisma with the manic's persuasiveness and intensity, and the effect is hypnotic. One of Napoleon's generals said: "This diabolical man had such power over me that I could not resist it." The chief surgeon of the army was not immune either: "[T]here was a sort of magnetic influence," he said, "which acted on an individual when ushered into his presence." Here is at least a partial explanation of how manic leaders can enlist rational people in their mad adventures.

Mania also enhanced Napoleon's considerable intelligence. Mania increases the speed at which a person thinks, as well as providing a plenitude of ideas for new projects and solutions to current problems. In its milder manifestations, mania increases creativity and resourcefulness. It also multiplies energy, enabling the manic to accomplish astonishing amounts of work. Napoleon thought and worked with extraordinary speed and with great agitation. If he started to dictate sitting in a chair, he soon became too excited to remain still and had to pace rapidly back and forth. When the brain is functioning at this abnormal rate, physical movement as well as thinking and speech are all speeded up. Pressured speech, as this rapid-fire talking is termed, is a symptom of mania, and Napoleon's speech was described as being "like a torrent." He spoke in such a rush that names would come out transposed. His secretaries could not begin to match his speed. To fill the time, he recalled, he would dictate "on different subjects, to four or five secretaries," and he could do this for several hours without pause. Even when he seemed to be resting, stretched out on a sofa, Napoleon was thinking furiously. As he put it, "When

I meditate, I'm in a state of agitation that is really painful. I'm like a girl having a baby."

While mania lasted, Napoleon's work day ran from fourteen to sixteen hours. If he stopped to eat, twenty minutes was as long as he would take before his energy propelled him back to work. There were many days when he refused to be interrupted even to dine. His doctor told him what doctors usually say to manic executives: he was working too hard. And it had the usual effect: none. Nothing could stop Napoleon but depression.

Napoleon's manic energy, of course, wore out the normal people who had to work with him. Often he would not let his legislators go home at the end of the day. He would shout: "Well, well, Citizens and Ministers, wake up! It's only two o'clock in the morning and you must earn the wages the French nation is paying you!" A fan of Napoleon once said, "God made Bonaparte, and then rested." His companion responded, "God should have rested a little earlier."

GENIUS AND BATTLE MANIA

The many benefits of mania combined to make Napoleon one of the most brilliant and effective generals in history. Time and again his daring and speed of response enabled him to defeat forces larger than his own. But his genius as a general existed only so long as he remained manic. His battle mania often commenced long before his soldiers took the field. The months of planning and of provisioning his armies engendered a manic state which intensified when the actual campaign was under way. During the fighting, Napoleon displayed a cluster of manic symptoms particularly advantageous for a military leader: excellent humor, optimism, enthusiasm, aggressiveness, confidence, daring, rapidity of thought and action, endless energy, little need for sleep, insensitivity to hunger or physical discomfort, and manic contagion. He often saw opportunities to take the enemy by surprise, then quickly marched his troops huge distances, his forces appearing when and where they were not expected. "My troops," he said, "moved as rapidly as my thoughts."

When on campaign, Napoleon's energy verged on the superhuman. One general reported: "On the days which preceded the battle he was constantly on horseback, reconnoitering the enemy's forces. Even in the night he used to visit the lines . . . and would tire out several horses in the space of a few hours." "I never comprehended how his body could endure such fatigue," wrote his valet Constant, "and yet he enjoyed almost continuously the most perfect health." On one occasion, Napoleon did not interrupt his activity for five days, even to change his clothes, and although he rode five horses to death, suffered no ill effects himself. On the contrary, war made Napoleon happy and flourishing. "After a trying six months' campaign," a witness said, "he would return stronger and healthier in appearance than before he left." There were no other generals in any army in Europe at that time who reacted with Napoleon's speed, or who could maintain his pace.

Manic contagion—the ability to inspire one's intense feelings in others—enabled Napoleon to impart his own confidence, enthusiasm, and aggressiveness to his troops. The Duke of Wellington, who ultimately defeated Napoleon at Waterloo, believed the Corsican's presence on the field was the equivalent of 40,000 soldiers.

The manic is oblivious of hunger, fatigue, and pain. And for a time at least, mania nullifies thoughts of danger and fears of dying. Fearless in battle, Napoleon was nearly captured more than once. It may be that many of those who earn medals for courage under fire are temporarily in the grip of mania. All this suggests that mania may have been preserved as part of the human inheritance because of its value in conflict.

Mania alone, of course, did not make Napoleon a wonder on the battlefield. But it was mania that lifted him far above the other able military men of his time who were closer to normalcy. It served him like a secret weapon, confounding the enemy time and again. Mania, therefore, was an essential condition for Napoleon's success, since his military victories were both the foundation for his rise to power and the means by which he extended his empire. Without the mania that came to Bonaparte in battle, the penniless Corsican artillery officer might have had a considerably more modest career.

INSTABILITY AND RAGE

Manic depression is rarely an unmitigated blessing. Mania may, without warning, turn into depression so incapacitating that the afflicted person can no longer function—as happened to Napoleon in Moscow, Dresden, and on other occasions. Manic depression can cause serious difficulties even for people who never experience the most extreme stages of the illness. Their sudden, unpredictable shifts of mood interfere with their plans. Napoleon in a mood of manic sociability would invite 800 guests to court, and then depression would prevent him from making an appearance. The change of mood can be startlingly abrupt and extreme. A secretary noted: "The very glance that had just been benign would suddenly dart lightning." Neither Napoleon nor anyone else could anticipate what his mood or behavior would be at any moment.

Others find manic depressives unreliable, often incomprehensible, and frequently unpleasant. Most puzzling to normal people is the fact that both depressive and manic episodes can strike inappropriately or without any external cause. More than once, Napoleon became manic before what looked like certain defeat. Equally strange to observers are the moods that occur at regular intervals. During some periods of his life, Napoleon's depressions arrived every morning but were gone by dinner.

While anger is not peculiar to the manic depressive, his anger requires little to ignite it and he often explodes into uncontrollable rages. The most trivial incident could set Napoleon off. Once he turned purple, screaming and stamping his feet because a piece of toothpick had become stuck between his teeth. On St. Helena, "he was yelling murder and assassination, raging, storming, swearing, and lashing out at all who came near him," a witness reported, because some cologne had gotten into his eye. And like other manic depressives, Napoleon could be physically violent. According to his valet, Constant, "The Emperor often broke his watch by throwing it at random . . . on any piece of furniture, leaving the scenes of his wrath looking as though bombs had detonated there." Bonaparte literally threw people out of rooms, although he was small for such exercise, and whipped servants who did not obey him quickly enough.

Their ferocious tempers make tyrannical manic depressives agonizing to work for. They terrify their employees, who live in constant anxiety, never knowing what to expect. Napoleon's petrified treasurer confessed, "I suffer from a pain in the stomach each time I have to make a report to the Emperor, and I lose my appetite completely for a few days." Another of Bonaparte's entourage observed, "No one was at ease in dealing with Napoleon, because no one could rely on a spirit of kindliness or indulgence. The smallest mishap, the slightest negligence sent him into fury." Besides being a source of torment to others, Napoleon's rages were also self-destructive in their personal and political consequences. Many of the people won over by Napoleon's charisma were later alienated by his tantrums.

The French emperor had greater emotional stability than the frequently frenzied Hitler and was more in touch with reality than the incredibly paranoid Stalin, but that is not saying much.

OVER THE EDGE

Like Hitler and Stalin, Napoleon became psychotic on occasion and developed delusions that were incorporated into his view of reality. As did Hitler and Stalin, Napoleon continued to cherish his fantastic beliefs even during those times when he saw the world most clearly. The result was that while he could be quite practical and deal effectively with the details of running an empire, his deepest motives for everything he did were quite irrational; important decisions were ultimately based on distortions of reality.

When he was manic, Napoleon's thinking was often distorted by grandiosity. He believed that he possessed supernatural powers, among them the ability to foretell everything that was going to take place. "Nothing ever happened to me that I did not foresee," he claimed. "I can divine everything in the future." Some of the delusions he developed on St. Helena combined grandiosity with manic optimism. He expected to be liberated by a change of government in England and planned to go to South America where, he promised, "I shall mold Latin America into a great empire." He thought that the laws of celestial mechanics had been abrogated to send him special signals in the form of a certain lucky star that appeared before all of his victories. According to Napoleon, this miraculous star also guaranteed his destiny to conquer and rule the world. This was a delusion combined with a visual hallucination, for he insisted he saw the star. "It has never abandoned me," Napoleon said in the years before he began to lose battles. "I see it on all occasions; it commands me to go forward, and it is a constant sign of my good fortune." The depressions of the last two years of his reign brought a new hallucination to Napoleon. He declared that fortune was deserting him and the harbinger of disaster that came to him was a spirit which he described as "the little red man." He "saw" this apparition frequently and claimed that it appeared every time things were about to go horribly wrong.

Hallucinations and persistent delusions are in themselves compelling evidence of psychosis. Napoleon's episodes of hyperactive mania, his stuporous depressions and suicide attempts confirm that he was severely ill with manic depression. The ill deserve compassion. But when the afflicted individual becomes a force in history, his illness transcends personal tragedy, for it may unleash on a helpless world all the evils that sanity reigns in.

14

Hitler's Emotion as a Political Force

What follows is a step-by-step survey of the various elements found in manic depression as they affected Adolf Hitler and supplied the propelling force in his rise to power. This chapter will also show the crippling effects of the illness, effects that made Hitler's success seem like a freak of politics.

One of the benefits of his illness that helped launch Hitler's political career was an overwhelming emotional force. Manic depressives simply have more intense emotion at their disposal than normal individuals. Hitler understood perfectly the power of emotion to persuade and inspire and control: "Only a storm of hot passion can turn the destinies of peoples," he said, "and he alone can arouse passion who bears it within himself." The impact of Hitler on susceptible individuals was extraordinary, as was his ability to move huge rallies to frenzy. One young German related how he felt the first time he heard Hitler speak: "I forgot everything but the man; then, glancing round, I saw that his magnetism was holding these thousands as I. Of course I was ripe for this experience . . . weary of disgust and disillusionment, a wanderer seeking a cause, a patriot without a channel for his patriotism, a yearner after the heroic without a hero. The intense will of the man, the passion of his sincerity seemed to flow from him into me. I experienced an exultation that could be likened only to a religious conversion. . . . I knew my search was ended. I had found myself, my leader, my cause."

With this extraordinary emotional force, Hitler could call on an equally startling persuasiveness—as can many manic depressives. He could cast a spell which made people believe he possessed, said an early devotee, "immense depths of sympathy and understanding. It was impossible to avoid being enveloped by him." Hitler was, unfortunately, too persuasive for his country's good. Rather than acknowledge unpleasant realities, he would persuade other more rational people that their gloomy reports were mistaken. Joachim von Ribbentrop recalled that officials who spent half an hour with Hitler "would support Adolf Hitler's point of view with the greatest conviction, although often it was the very opposite of what they had meant to tell him."

Although it seems incredible that someone so filled with hate could ever appear to be likable, Hitler's arsenal of manic assets included charm, and this helped him to influence people. "When he was out to win someone over or to get something out of somebody," Ribbentrop observed, "he could be extra-ordinarily charming and persuasive."

Hitler was not a hyperactive ruler like Napoleon, but the manic energy he had when he campaigned was a considerable advantage—as it is for many politicians. It also occasionally assisted Hitler after his rise to power. At such times the ordinarily valetudinarian Hitler duplicated the freedom from physical need that Napoleon enjoyed during battle mania. "Astonishing are the explosions of his . . . sudden activity," Dr. Hermann Rauschning, president of the Danzig parliament, said. "Then he neither tires nor hungers; he lives with morbid energy that enables him to do almost miraculous things."

Most delusions are harmful to those who are misled by them; but one, the grandiose conviction that they have a special destiny, is the cornerstone of the careers of many people who become highly successful despite disadvantageous origins. Without that initially unproven faith in themselves, most people are unlikely to take the chances, make the sacrifices, and expend the effort needed to surpass the competition. It was certainly so in Hitler's case. In 1919 he developed the grandiose delusion that he, alone of all mankind, understood all of human history and what he "understood" was that he would make Germany great. It was such delusions that enabled Hitler to fight his way to the leadership of Germany. Alfred Rosenberg, an early supporter, recorded that from the beginning Hitler had "a fanatical belief in his own mission which, toward the end, actually became incomprehensible."

Hitler was also sustained by a particular delusions he shared with Napoleon—that he was invulnerable, at least until he had accomplished his mission on earth: "I believe very deeply that destiny has selected me for the German nation. So long as I am needed by the people, so long as I am responsible for the life of the Reich, I shall live." This delusion must have been a comfort to the führer when the bombs were falling on Berlin.

HITLER'S HANDICAPS

Manic depression gave Hitler far fewer benefits than it gave to Napoleon, and was much more damaging. To make matters worse, almost every beneficial symptom Hitler had was ultimately nullified by a detrimental symptom.

The downside to all Hitler's emotional power was that his thinking was clouded by the intensity of his emotions. "His political common sense," Alfred Rosenberg observed, "was frequently derailed by his sudden outbursts of passion." His uncontrollable and radically unstable emotions were also a great impediment to the efficient operation of the government. "Everything depended on the way he was feeling, his moods," noted Otto Dietrich. Hitler was adverse to schedules; necessary meetings of government departments were suspended for months, even for years. The führer seldom wrote out his orders or gave them in any predictable fashion, but simply announced them, as inspiration moved him, to the person standing nearest. Hitler even advocated that everyone adopt his chaotic style. "Trust your instincts, your feelings, whatever you like to call them."

Governing by impulse is characteristic of a manic depressive whether he be a head of state or the Chief Executive Officer of a corporation, for the manic is ruled by his impulses. A tyrant's entourage learns to maneuver around the despot's moods. Hitler's associates put off executing orders they did not like until he forgot about them or took advantage of his moods to elicit the orders that they wanted. The drawbacks of government by mood and whim eventually became ruinous. During his depressions Hitler was so indecisive that even urgent matters had to wait and serious problems became insoluble ones.

Hitler's high-voltage emotions worked for him at mass rallies, but they often sabotaged him when he spoke to individuals. This could be inconvenient to say the least. One individual who came away from his interviews with Hitler convinced that the führer was "a quasi-madman," was André François-Poncet, France's pre-war ambassador to Germany. "At the beginning of the conversation he seemed not to listen," the ambassador noted.

> Then suddenly, as though a hand had released a lever, he would burst forth into a harangue, uttered in shrill, excited, choleric tones. His arguments, gathering speed and volume, came more abundantly . . . and he roared and thundered as though addressing thousands of listeners. . . . It was useless to seek to interrupt him or to protest. . . . These "fits" might last ten minutes or even three-quarters of an hour. Then suddenly . . . it was as though his batteries had run dry [and] he relapsed into inertia. . . . When in this state . . . he would hesitate, ask for time to think things over, procrastinate.

Hitler, in this instance, shot out of a depression into a brief manic state, then subsided into depressive passivity once more. Both mania and depression reached such extremes in him that he developed two separate and opposing personalities, each with its own standards of behavior. When manic Hitler boasted about being the world's best liar, "the greatest actor in Europe." "Treaties exist," Hitler said, "for the purpose of being broken at the most convenient moment." However, when he descended from his elation, he thought of himself as the soul of probity. "Have I ever in my life told a lie?" he once asked in perfect seriousness.

In one mood Hitler ordered the extermination of all senile people, mental and tubercular patients, and those suffering from birth defects. In another he remembered his secretaries' birthdays and helped people who had been kind to him when he was poor. "When I think about it," Hitler said, "I realize that I'm extraordinarily humane." He fed birds and insisted that restaurants try to reduce the pain of lobsters being boiled alive. But he often carried a whip and used it. A friend recalled seeing Hitler whip his dog "like a madman . . . an animal about which he had said a moment previously that he could not live without." To attractive young women Hitler showed what one of them described as a "strange tenderness and appealing helplessness." Albert Speer, who saw the other side of Hitler, summed him up as "a ruthless and mankind-hating nihilist." So violently dissimilar were Hitler's personalities that, said Dietrich, those who had seen only one phase "could not possibly imagine what the other Hitler was like." When mildly depressed, Hitler was modest, sympathetic, sentimental, and lachrymose. In mania, his characteristics, according to Dr. Rauschning, were "contemptuousness, arrogance, brutality, vanity."

No one, least of all Hitler himself, ever knew when he would shift from one personality to its extreme opposite, which he could do in the blink of an eye. Hitler's incalculable and frightening shifts of personality increased his isolation from the people whose support was crucial to him, and from reality as well.

The charm and persuasiveness that were Hitler's gifts from mania ultimately did him little good, for he had a number of nasty manic behaviors that corroded what friendly relationships he managed to develop. He often made fun of people, taunting them with barbed jibes under the guise of being playful. He undermined trust by embroidering statements with extravagant exaggerations or by lying outright. One of the few occasions when Hitler was entirely honest was when he warned one of his generals, "Those who boast most loudly that they know my thoughts, to such people I lie even more."

The manic drive that made Hitler a formidable campaigner often interfered with tasks that required concentration. He found it difficult to read a book through—he would scan a few pages, then drop the book, saying that he knew what was in it anyway. It was difficult for him to take in information from any source: the distractibility of mania prevented him from listening to people even when he was willing to do so. "It was almost impossible to keep Hitler concentrated on one point," a witness recalled. "His quick mind would run away . . . or his attention would be distracted by the sudden discovery of a newspaper, and he would stop and read it avidly, or he would interrupt your carefully prepared report with a long speech as though you were an audience." Hitler's manic impatience not only preserved his ignorance, it also guaranteed that he would not take the time to give a second thought to his decisions.

Dr. Rauschning noted that Hitler's impulses "must be feverishly achieved and immediately got rid of."

As in his youth, when he bored his friend Kubizek with long diatribes, Hitler continued, when führer, to give endless manic monologues that usually lasted past midnight and sometimes until morning. Driven by pressure of speech, he either did not realize or did not care that he told the same stories and jokes over and over. Sometimes his manic impulsiveness and compulsion to talk betrayed him into spilling secrets of state.

More serious still were Hitler's terrible fits of rage. Many manics are unable to bear criticism, contradiction, or frustration. Hitler could not tolerate any of the three and his response could be terrifying. "Almost anything," Dr. Rauschning recalled, "might suddenly inflame his wrath and his hatred." The suggestion that Hitler had whistled a tune incorrectly, a newspaper's omission to mention the death of a favorite opera singer on the front page, a valet forgetting to bring his favorite mineral water—all sufficed to infuriate the führer.

Dr. Rauschning described a typical Hitlerian explosion: "He scolded in high, shrill tones, stamped his feet, and banged his fist on tables and walls. He foamed at the mouth, panting and stammering in uncontrollable fury. . . . He was an alarming sight, his hair disheveled, his eyes fixed, his face distorted and purple." Paranoia added a lethal quality to Hitler's rages. They "occurred whenever events took a course different from that which Hitler had willed and predicted," noted his press chief. "When he was in such a state, trivial blunders and oversights would be branded damnable crimes. Death penalties or the concentration camp were . . . often the result of his uncontrollable rages."

Hitler was better known for his manic behavior than for what he did when depressed, perhaps because in his depressed states he often retreated into solitude. He refused to see people, or ran off to his residence at Berchtesgaden, where he walked the countryside alone. His depressions were severe enough, however, to be completely disabling. Dr. Rauschning observed that Hitler's depressions made the führer feel "humiliated," "weak-willed," "inert and apathetic," as well as irritable and indecisive. Hitler would collapse in "convulsions of weeping" or remain locked in long silences, Dr. Rauschning reported, "picking his teeth abominably."

These depressions brought in their train a set of fantastic beliefs quite different from those with which mania deceived Hitler. However, he accepted these, too, apparently unaware that his depressive delusions contradicted his manic ones. For example, while mania made Hitler feel invulnerable, depression made him phobic. He was afraid of infectious diseases and kept washing his hands. His phobias included bodies of water, horses, and the moon. Depression also brought frequent attacks of anxiety. "He wakes at night with convulsive shrieks," Dr. Rauschning wrote. "He shouts for help. He sits on the edge of his bed, as if unable to stir. He shakes with fear, making the whole bed vibrate. He shouts confused, totally unintelligible phrases." Hitler tried to find relief from his stuporous depressions by taking, at various times, vitamins, cocaine, amphetamines, and preparations made from the sexual glands of male animals, these last intended also to restore potency.

Hypochondria is another symptom of depression that had a considerable effect on Hitler's life. He often took his own pulse and would exclaim, with tears in his eyes, "If only my health were good!" He interpreted stomach cramps as symptoms of cancer. At one point he was taking twenty-eight different drugs.

The symptoms which give indisputable evidence that Hitler had reached the worst stages of his illness were his suicide attempts, ten of which appear in the surviving data, and the hallucinations that occurred in both his manic and depressive states. Chapter 5 recounted a manic auditory hallucination that occurred at the end of World War I, when Hitler was told by imaginary voices to save Germany. A depressive visual hallucination took place during the 1930s. Dr. Rauschning describes it:

> He stood swaying in his room looking wildly about him. "He! He! He's been here!" he gasped. . . . Sweat streamed down his face. Suddenly he began to reel off figures, and odd words and broken phrases, entirely devoid of sense. . . . Then he stood quite still, only his lips moving. . . . Then he suddenly broke out: "There, there! in the corner! Who's that?" He stamped and shrieked in the familiar way. He was shown that there was nothing out of the ordinary in the room and at last he grew calm.

DEADLY DELUSIONS

The symptoms of manic depression discussed so far had their most profound effect on Hitler himself, on the people around him, and on the government he led. However, there were other symptoms—delusions—whose impact was felt far beyond the borders of Germany. World history would have been far different had Hitler been oriented in reality or subject to different delusions than the ones that drove him, especially had he not suffered from the paranoid hatreds that spurred him to genocide.

To protect himself from his personal devils, Hitler created his Aryan angels, whom he defined as the true Germans, whether they were found in Germany or elsewhere. He shared with many Germans of his day the misconception that Aryans were a race of genetically similar people: blond, blue-eyed, muscular—a description which, incidentally, excluded Hitler himself and many members of the Nazi party.

Aryans are not a race but rather a genetically diverse group whose common characteristic is that they speak Indo-European languages. Nonetheless, Hitler and many other Germans erected a complex delusional system on their foundation of fantasy. "All the human culture, all the results of art, science, and technology that we see before us today, are almost exclusively the creative product of the Aryan," Hitler proclaimed. Rather than learn something about history, Hitler relied on his delusions to explain everything. "The racial question gives the key not only to world history, but to all human culture," he said. The Aryan was the only "good race" and those who did not belong to it should have no more rights than livestock. "All who are not of good race in this world are chaff," he said repeatedly. He made a religion of racial prejudice. "There is only one holiest right, and this right is at the same time the holiest obligation, to wit: to see that the blood is preserved pure . . . to produce images of the Lord and not monstrosities halfway between man and ape." His anti-Semitism, Hitler insisted, was divinely inspired: "I believe that I am acting in accordance with the will of the Almighty Creator: by defending myself against the Jew, I am fighting for the work of the Lord."

If the so-called Aryans were the angels in Hitler's Manichean world of good and evil, the Jews were the demonic adversary. As early as 1922, when asked about his intentions toward Jews, Hitler went into a manic tirade and yelled, "[T]he destruction of the Jews will be my first and most important job. . . . I shall have gallows after gallows erected. . . . Then the Jews will be hanged one after another and they will stay hanging until they stink." Shortly after seizing power, Hitler proclaimed that he would remove the Jews from Europe and then go on to "the elimination of the Jews altogether." Not only was Hitler, for once, utterly sincere, but also such pronouncements were politically useful in anti-Semitic Germany—although many decent Germans would have boggled at the thought that Hitler really intended to follow through with the Holocaust.

The paranoia that inspired Hitler's hatred of Jews was unmistakable at a birthday party given for him in 1923. Admirers filled his apartment with gifts and fancy cakes. He warned a visiting friend not to eat anything there. "Don't forget," he said, "this building belongs to a Jew and it's child's play to let poison trickle down the walls in order to dispose of an enemy." Hitler's paranoid delusions about Jews were a factor in his determination to conquer the world. "The struggle for world domination," he said, "will be fought entirely between us, between Germans and Jews. All else is facade and illusion. Behind England stands Israel, and behind France, and behind the United States. Even when we have driven the Jew out of Germany, he remains our world enemy."

Hitler's entire view of reality was, like Stalin's and to some degree Napoleon's, filtered through a dark, distorting lens of paranoia. Eventually, paranoia left him completely isolated: "I can trust no one," he said. The führer did not confine his paranoid suspicions to his entourage. He also assailed diplomats with wild accusations. His paranoia, whatever it may have contributed to foreign relations, was decidedly detrimental to the war effort. Hitler developed unjustified suspicions about many of his most capable officers and got rid of them.

The Jews were not the only group that Hitler feared as a menace and his paranoia fostered some strikingly original delusions. "France," he exclaimed, "is by far the most terrible enemy. This people, which is basically becoming more and more negrified, constitutes in its tie with the aims of the Jewish world domination an enduring danger for the existence of the white race in Europe." He decided that Christianity had no genuine ethics because it developed from the "first Jewish-Communistic cell." Among other grave threats that Hitler identified were Catholics and especially Jehovah's Witnesses. He disposed of the latter by shipping them to death camps. Hitler ordered the extermination of other categories of people, both within Germany and wherever German forces were in control. Besides people whom he considered mentally or physically defective, he wanted all Gypsies and all Communists annihilated. Also on his enemies list were people of any nationality who were skiers, hunters, journalists, judges, poets, smokers, Freemasons, and anyone who was not a vegetarian. He even hated a particular segment of the German people—the German middle class. "We never know which is greater in the bourgeois world, their imbecility, weakness, and cowardice, or their deep-dyed corruption. It is truly a class doomed by Fate, but unfortunately, however, it is dragging a whole nation with it into the abyss." As always, Hitler gave others the credit for his own disasters, in this instance blaming the German middle class for the collapse of the nation.

Napoleon was a champion of death because his ambitions cost millions of lives. To Napoleon's lust for conquest, Hitler added a new malevolent design to exterminate an entire people. As will be seen in chapter 17, manic depression played the key role in making Hitler both a tyrant and a genocide.

15

Stalin's Darkness

The shoemaker's son showed, even as a boy, streaks of the manic arrogance and ambition that would keep him grasping at power until no more was to be had. Had Stalin not been a manic depressive, he would have lacked the drive and self-confidence necessary to claw his way to leadership of the Soviet Union. However, unlike Napoleon and Hitler, the Georgian was predominantly a depressive for the first five decades of his life. His brother-in-law, Stanislav Redens, described him as a "sullen man." Before he was fifty, Stalin had periods of mania, such as at Tsaritsyn in 1918 (see chapter 8), which prefigured the man he would become once he had absolute supremacy. But depression left permanent stains on Stalin's habits and character.

Depression also stamped Stalin's political personality. He lacked the magnetism of the manic. He never became a thundering orator like Hitler; he never developed Napoleon's and Hitler's hypnotic powers of persuasion. Trotsky mentioned "his complete inability to catch fire . . . to conjure a vital bond between himself and his audience, to arouse an audience to its better self. Unable to catch fire himself, he was incapable of inflaming others." Since Stalin could not inspire others to follow him, he became a leader by scheming and through subterfuge, and relied primarily on terror to exert control. Gray as a rainy winter was his style, even when he could command the wealth of the tsars. Stalin lacked the manic's *joie de vivre*. He made life dreary for himself and, except when he was carried away by mania, dreary for everyone who lived under his rule.

LIFE IN AN OLD COAT

The depressive often looks like a refugee from a rummage sale. He deprives himself of pleasures he can afford and fails to enjoy even the little that he allows himself. Thus it was with Stalin. The Georgian plumbed the depths of sartorial squalor. He wore an unadorned military tunic over baggy trousers and top boots. He had, says Svetlana, "a short, strange-looking fur coat with squirrel on the inside and reindeer on the outside, which he started wearing soon after the Revolution. Stalin went on wearing it . . . to the end of his days," which was thirty-six years later.

He rarely went to the several houses he acquired, staying for the most part at his Kuntsevo bungalow. Even after making improvements in that structure, Stalin confined himself to a fraction of the house. He lived only in one room, which became office, dining room, parlor, and bedroom, though it contained only a couch for a bed. His Kremlin office was furnished only with a long table and some wooden chairs. For decor there were images of Marx, Engels, Lenin, and two Imperial Russian generals.

As his daughter Svetlana commented, "My father never cared about possessions." Stalin, however, took care to place himself on numerous government payrolls and after he died, drawers were found stuffed with unopened pay envelopes. He had manic spurts of greed but, like a true depressive, denied himself full use of what he had acquired. And like many depressives, he was stingy and hated to spend money.

Self-deprivation could pass into self-punishment. During the earlier part of his life, before power made him manic and grandiose, Stalin appeared to dislike himself, as depressives often do, and had at least one self-destructive episode. While he was incarcerated in the Baku prison, he once asked a cellmate: "Do you have a craving for blood?" Without waiting for an answer, Stalin withdrew a knife that he had hidden in his boot, pulled up the leg of his trousers, and plunged the blade into the exposed skin, saying, "There's blood for you!" The American journalist Eugene Lyons reported: "All those who have been close to him and dared to speak afterwards have remarked on the symptoms of his profound feelings of inferiority."

THE PERPETUAL OUTSIDER

When not in his manic periods, Stalin had the depressive's discomfort with strangers. The approach of a crowd come to welcome him with cheers and bouquets set his face twitching. He was a very private dictator. Khrushchev complained: "Stalin separated himself from the people and never went anywhere. . . . The last time he visited a village was in January 1928." Stalin generally avoided being seen by the public except on obligatory holidays.

Depressives, although they tend to withdraw from people or drive them away, often complain of loneliness. They fear being abandoned. They are uneasy with people, but they need distraction from their misery and, at times, try to avoid being alone. This is what Stalin did in his later years. As he had by then estranged himself from those relatives he had not killed, he relied on his political entourage to ward off his depressions. Khrushchev testified: "He needed people around him all the time. When he woke up in the morning, he would immediately summon us, either inviting us to a film show or starting a conversation which could have been finished in two minutes. But he stretched it so that we could stay with him. . . . The main thing was to occupy Stalin's time so he would not suffer loneliness. He was depressed by loneliness and he feared it."

Fear is a prominent symptom of many depressions, and may run the gamut from anxiety to phobia. Stalin was afraid of many things, including the streets of Moscow, into which he never ventured in his later years. His fear of crowds and of strangers may have been phobias heightened by paranoia. Two of his problems, however, were simply phobias: his fears of heights and of flying. The meetings with Churchill and Roosevelt were held in Teheran and Potsdam because Stalin could reach those cities by rail.

THE VULNERABLE "MAN OF STEEL"

A moderate degree of mania makes people resilient and resourceful in crises. Depression has the opposite effect. Stalin frequently became depressed when events went against him, and he reacted badly to stress throughout his life. According to Trotsky, Stalin would abandon what he was doing when anything happened that lowered his self-esteem: "Whenever he feels himself ignored or neglected, he is inclined to turn his back upon developments as well as upon people, creep into a corner, moodily pull on his pipe."

Stalin had difficulty coping with even minor domestic upsets. When he was left for a few moments in charge of his infant son Yakov, he responded to the baby's cry by puffing smoke in his face and putting the pipe in the infant's mouth. The baby howled at this treatment. Angered by his son's reaction, Stalin yelled, "There's a blackguard for you! He's not a good Bolshevik!" The furious father threw his baby back into the crib and, says a witness, "The whole evening had been ruined for him . . . until he went to bed, he pottered about, whining peevishly and finding fault with everything."

Years of triumph and mania brought no improvement in Stalin's ability to function under pressure. Unfortunately for his country, the dictator's depressive behavior had historic consequences. His inability to confront unpleasant or frightening situations was almost fatal to the USSR when Germany was preparing to invade, and he collapsed when the invasion took place. Stalin lacked the manic's courage. Bloodshed excited him, but he preferred to observe riots and battles from a safe distance. Stalin easily succumbed to anxiety and would abandon enterprises that met with resistance. He did so when the Americans countered his blockade of Berlin with the airlift.

Depression makes people avoid whatever task appears discouraging or onerous to them. Khrushchev saw this behavior in the last years of the Georgian's life. "Stalin often failed for months to take up some unusually important problems, concerning the life of the party and of the state, whose solution could not be postponed."

STALIN ON A SEESAW

Intense emotionality was one of the many signs of manic depression that Stalin exhibited from time to time. Churchill saw him wiping tears from his eyes when a baritone at the Bolshoi sang ballads about exile in Siberia.

Stalin also exhibited the rapid alteration of feelings common to the manic depressive. Trotsky found him "moody to the point of capriciousness." Even when Stalin made an effort to appear genial in the presence of foreigners, "opposition to his will," noted a British translator, "could at any moment change the atmosphere to one of gloom and hostility." Changes of mood could even lead Stalin to release people from prison. A man he had expelled from the party and sent to a labor camp was released for no reason, as he had been imprisoned for no reason. On seeing him, Stalin asked in a friendly way where he had been keeping himself. Shortly thereafter, Stalin made his ex-prisoner ambassador to Romania.

Stalin's working hours, like Hitler's and Napoleon's, suggest that he had a twenty-four-hour mood cycle which made him most manic in the evening. His working day began an hour before noon. He usually saw foreign dignitaries in the evening. If he entertained them, he would do so from ten until five or six the following morning. When no foreigners were visiting, he regularly invited his associates to "working" dinners during which he sometimes became elated and uproarious. The dictator also showed signs of an annual mood cycle, being more benign in the summer and more lethal in the winter. He generally alternated between periods of high political activity and periods of quiet.

TWO STALINS

Most descriptions of the depressive Stalin refer to the dictator's early years while descriptions of the manic Stalin refer to the man who ruled the Soviet Union. The young Georgian revolutionary had an air of depression about him.

One of the friends of his youth called him "a gloomy, unsociable man, who never perhaps in his whole life laughed or smiled except out of the side of his mouth." When the struggle for power was won, Stalin began to display a manic personality even to foreigners. George Bernard Shaw, on a visit to the Soviet Union in 1931, found Stalin witty: "Unlike other dictators, Stalin has an irrepressible sense of humor." Lord Beaverbrook noted: "He is always ready to laugh, quick to see a joke, and willing to make one." Milovan Djilas, on a trip to see the dictator in 1944, also encountered the manic side of his personality: "Stalin had a sense of humor—a rough humor, self-assured, but not entirely without finesse and depth."

Depression slowed Stalin's thought and his speech in his earlier years. "We knew him as a slow and plodding thinker," reported Alexander Barmine, a Soviet bureaucrat. "Stalin speaks in a slow monotone which is tiring to the ear." Barmine also noted that "at Politburo and Central Committee meetings during Lenin's lifetime both before and after the Revolution, he used to sit apart, sulky and silent, unable to participate in the rapid fire of ideas." At times, minutes would pass before Stalin responded to something said to him. Depression can noticeably reduce the speed of thought. In contrast to the slow-witted, sulky, younger Stalin, Djilas saw an older one whose "reactions were quick and acute."

Depression diminishes people's desire to speak. In the first half of his life, Stalin had little to say. When he spoke, his voice expressed a depressive apathy. Trotsky observed this at meetings: "He would force himself to utter sentences with great difficulty, without tonality, without warmth, without emphasis." But mania made Stalin talkative and even eloquent. "His Russian vocabulary was rich," Djilas commented, "his manner of expression very vivid and plastic, and replete with Russian proverbs and sayings." The dictator spent many nights after World War II chatting and arguing for hours with his guests at his vacation home on the Black Sea. He became a tireless raconteur—to the distress of Khrushchev who recalled "interminable, agonizing dinners" listening to Stalin's stories.

In the early days, Barmine said, "What held my attention . . . was Stalin's amazing patience." The "amazing patience" was actually the product of the depressive's mental lethargy. As Stalin's mind took on a manic speed, the patience vanished. Djilas noted, "He was no friend of long explanations." In his later years, the dictator lacked the patience to listen to his own applause and frequently cut it short.

MANIC MASKS

Mania can make people warm, generous, loving, and altruistic. Unfortunately, there was little in Stalin of the benign side of mania, except for a brief period when his daughter Svetlana was a child. In those few years, he was playful and loving, but only with her. He wrote to her: "I give my little sparrow a big hug," "I give you a kiss," "I'm glad you haven't forgotten your little papa." He signed his letters to her: "the poor peasant J. Stalin." According to a game he had established, she sent him orders to which he would respond, "I submit" or "I obey." Svetlana would threaten to complain about her father to the cook, and he would plead: "Spare me! If you complain to the cook, it will be all over wtih me!" He was affectionate when at home and often sent packages of fancy fruits when away.

Stalin was genuinely charming to his daughter but, for the most part, such charm as he displayed was play-acting. Many manics make a practice of dissembling and manipulation; Stalin went further than most. He created an entirely fictitious personality that he exhibited to visiting foreigners and to the Soviet public. On kindergarten walls hung an obligatory photograph of the leader holding a six-year-old girl who had just given him a bouquet. Later he ordered the death of her father. He played the unassuming, kindly father of all Russia while attributing the autocratic rule his people suffered to the actions of government ministries and committees, judicial and legislative bodies.

In his later years, Stalin liked to boast about his abilities and, like many manics, embellished his stories outrageously. "It's hard to say why Stalin felt he had to lie," Khrushchev later mused. "He must have had some inner urge."

This habitual mendacity was a hallmark of Stalin's rule. Of our three dictators he was the most consistent political liar; indeed, it would be difficult to find his equal anywhere. Stalin invariably applauded himself as the moderate ruler of a free and democratic state when he was inflicting some new form of repression on his country. He commended collective leadership, but, says Khrushchev, "A 'proposal' from Stalin was a God-given command, and you don't haggle about what God tells you to do—you just offer thanks and obey." Stalin exclaimed, "God forbid that we should be infected with the disease of fearing the truth," while at the same time controlling all education and information media and jamming foreign broadcasts. He praised legality as he broke the laws and castrated the judicial system. He gave the people what he called "the most democratic constitution in the world," and made it a dead letter.

MANIC MOMENTUM

In his earlier years, when depression predominated, Stalin was not remarkable for speed or energy except during rare manic spurts. Instead of slowing further as he entered middle age, however, he developed a manic tempo. When working, he would deliver long monologues while pacing back and forth, and tolerated no interruptions. Like Napoleon, Stalin paced while dictating. He would walk around briskly as people delivered oral reports. He also left his chair during Politburo meetings and marched up and down. When Djilas visited the manic Stalin, restlessness was a main characteristic the Yugoslav noticed: "He was not quiet for a moment. He toyed with his pipe . . . or drew circles with a blue pencil . . . and he kept turning his head this way and that while he fidgeted in his seat."

In his later years Stalin, like Hitler, adopted a manically impulsive style of governing; his colleagues learned to stand by with paper and pencil at the ready, exactly as was done with Hitler. Orders were issued at all times of the day and night, even at banquets and bacchanals. The Georgian's sudden inspirations built a canal between the Don and Volga rivers and divided postwar Germany into eastern and western parts. Stalin often cut meetings short or changed the purpose of the meeting as the mood moved him. Since everything depended on Stalin's moods, the Politburo held no regular, official meetings. Without warning, the dictator would arrive in Moscow and summon the Politburo members, usually to meet in the Kremlin movie theater. "We would watch movies and talk about various matters between reels," Khrushchev recalled. "As a rule, when the movie ended, Stalin would suggest, 'Well, let's go get something to eat, why don't we?' . . . When we got to the dacha, the 'session' continued, if you can call it a session." As there were no regular meetings of the Central Committee, the Politburo, and the Presidium, the government's highest bodies, "the government virtually ceased to function," Khrushchev added.

The dictator's whims determined who had access to him, and that could not be predicted from one day to the next. Moreover, people could remain out of favor for indefinite periods that sometimes were terminated by arrest and execution.

SEX AND OBSCENITY

Exhibitionism and other kinds of offensive sexual behavior may appear in the more intense manic states. A friend from the Caucasus who was accustomed to Stalin's being "foul-mouthed," was shocked to hear him singing obscene songs in "the presence of . . . highly moral women." Stalin would use the chamber pot in his office while aides, female secretaries, or visitors were present.

A voracious sexual appetite is a common sign of mania. Stalin's manic personality emerged during his second marriage. Like Napoleon, Stalin became promiscuous as he shifted from a primarily depressive personality to a manic one. He had intercourse with the adolescent daughter of a colleague, Lazar Kaganovich. Stalin often ordered his drinking companions to bring women to his office. Some of the women were provided by K. V. Pauker, who began as Stalin's valet and eventually was made security chief for the Kremlin. Pauker also supplied pornographic movies from abroad. Sometimes Stalin picked up women at drunken parties given by his old companion Abel Yenukidze. During his marriage to Nadya, Stalin had a mistress, Yolka Andreyevna, who gave birth to one of Stalin's sons.

Khrushchev and Svetlana both wrote of a young woman who moved into the house after Nadya's death. Khrushchev recorded: "I remember seeing a young, beautiful Georgian woman around. Somebody said she was Svetlana's tutor. . . . One day she just disappeared." In 1938 Stalin began a three-year-long affair with a typist during which she bore him a daughter, whom he placed in an orphanage. While this woman, Anya Markovna Chernikova, was with him, he had affairs with actresses, ballet dancers, and Kremlin employees, occasionally making a threesome with Anya. When he was over 60, Stalin took a twenty-three-year-old mistress, Yevgeniya Pavlovna Movshina. This liaison, during which there were other women as well, lasted six years. It terminated when Stalin found Yevgeniya in bed with another man. He beat them both until they were bloody, then called Beria, who had them shot in Lubyanka Prison. For a while Stalin had a succession of teenage girls who came to his office, where dancing nude was one of the activities demanded of them. Sadism may have been part of the entertainment he required. Some of the girls were observed leaving Stalin's office in tears. Stalin took another mistress in 1952, Lyda Mikhailovna Vavryna, who became pregnant not long before Stalin died.

A GROWING THIRST

Stalin's alcoholism was probably inherited, as was his manic depression; each disorder must have exacerbated the ill effects of the other. Stalin was not aware of either illness, although he knew he was fond of alcohol. By his own account, his heavy drinking began while he was a revolutionary in exile in Siberia. Khrushchev quotes a reminiscence from Stalin's first exile: "Stalin used to say, 'There were some nice fellows among the criminal convicts during my exile. I hung around mostly with the criminals. I remember we used to stop at the saloons in town. We'd . . . drink up every kopek we had.' "

Rosa Kaganovich, the woman who took the place of Stalin's second wife, confirmed that the dictator's abuse of alcohol began well before World War II. She stated that he had a half pint of vodka with breakfast, another at lunch, and a bottle of wine at dinner. Once the war was over, Stalin gave drunken parties every two or three days. The dictator's guests were impressed with the amount of alcohol their host consumed and wondered how he had acquired his drinking habits. Khrushchev recalled the dictator's own explanation that his father had made him a drinker literally as an infant. "My father," Stalin said, "used to dip his finger in a glass of wine and let me suck on it. He was teaching me to drink even when I was still in the cradle."

Stalin insisted that his guests keep up with his own consumption of alcohol. At Stalin's dinners, Khrushchev states, "there were often serious drinking bouts. . . . I remember Beria, Malenkov, and Mikoyan had to ask the waitress to pour them colored water instead of wine because they couldn't keep up with Stalin's drinking." He added that "when Stalin realized he had been deceived he fumed with anger and raised a terrible uproar." The dictator wanted to be the one who played tricks.

CRUEL HUMOR

Like many irritable manics, Stalin was critical and sarcastic, made fun of the people around him, and enjoyed cruel practical jokes. "For some reason he found the humiliation of others very amusing." Khrushchev noted. He also vividly recalled when his own turn came. "I remember once Stalin made me dance the 'Gopak' before some top party officials. I had to squat down on my haunches and kick out my heels, which frankly wasn't very easy for me. But I did it and I tried to keep a pleasant expression on my face." Stalin was quite capable of humiliating even his daughter once she had left childhood. After World War I, at a dinner given for twelve Soviet marshals, Stalin said in his daugher's presence, "Well, my friends, I bet you don't know who's fucking her now." He laughed as she ran out of the room.

GEORGIAN RAGE

Stalin's temper, like that of many manics, was both unpredictable and ferocious, as Khrushchev attested: "It was as though the devil himself held a string attached to Stalin's main nerve, and no one knew when the devil would give the string a jerk, sending Stalin into one of his fits of rage."

As mania intensifies, so does irritability and the propensity for violence. Stalin became known for violence when he was a young revolutionary. He would lose control during arguments with party members, cursing them and throwing objects such as stools. When he was married to his first wife, Kato, Stalin's brutality was witnessed by a man with whom they were living: "Scum, that's what he is," said his fellow revolutionary. "Kato was pregnant then, and he used to curse her in the most disgusting way. And kick her in the belly."

There was no improvement in Stalin's temper during his second marriage. He threw food out the window if he was bored with what had been cooked, and his daughter recalled him slamming a telephone against the wall because it had been giving a busy signal. Often Stalin's violence sprang from nowhere. When he found a large mirror in his new Kremlin apartment he said, "What's a mirror here for?" and kicked it to pieces. He began beating and kicking his sons when they were small. On one occasion a visting friend tried to restore calm. Stalin ordered him, in the vilest terms, to get out. Their father's ferocious battering did not abate as the boys grew older, and he turned on his daughter, too.

PERSONAL PARANOIA

Stalin's obsession with power was equaled only by his paranoia, and the two augmented each other. The more power he had, the greater was his fear that someone would wrest it from him. Stalin sought security in having absolute control over everyone else, but instead, his success made him feel more vulnerable. It was a vicious circle that tightened into a noose from which he could not free himself. Once his power over the Soviet Union was absolute, and the threat of Hitler was gone, Stalin could not rest until he had buttressed the USSR with the nations of Eastern Europe. Then he worried about maintaining his iron control over them.

Stalin's attempts to assure his supremacy and personal safety never ceased. Wary of doctors, he took over his own medication. In a fever of suspicion, he was about to launch another bloody purge when he died. His paranoia may have been the ultimate cause of Stalin's death if, as it appears, his intended victims killed him to preserve their own lives. The tyrant was, indavertently, his own severest judge, for he condemned himself to a life sentence of terror and a death sentence by assassination. His bloody policies brought upon himself the very end they were designed to prevent.

Stalin's paranoia extended to his own family. He believed his older son Yakov had committed treason by being captured by the Germans. The enraged father declared, "in Hitler's camps there are no Russian prisoners of war, only Russian traitors, and we shall do away with them when the war is over." He decided that Yakov's Jewish wife had conspired in the betrayal and had her arrested by the NKVD. When Yakov heard that his father had accused him of treason, he committed suicide by running into the electrified fence of the prison camp. In 1943, in a fleeting benevolent mood, Stalin decided that Yakov had conducted himself honorably as a prisoner and released Yakov's wife.

The dictator also concluded that Nadya, his second wife, had been a traitor to him because she criticized his persecutions. The same befell several of Stalin's male in-laws, who were also unwise enough to intercede for the victims of Stalin's paranoia. "The only thing they accomplished by it," Svetlana reported, "was loss of access to my father and total forfeiture of his trust. When he saw each of them for the last time, it was as if he were parting with someone who was no longer a friend, with someone, in fact, who was already an enemy." Five years after Nadya's murder or suicide, whichever it was, Stalin commenced the destruction of all those close to her, his customary procedure with families of his victims. Nadya's godfather, Abel Yenukidze, was arrested and shot. Stanislav Redens, her sister's first husband, was shot. Her brother, Pavel, died officially of heart failure but this was a disguised murder. Pavel's wife was forbidden to see Stalin's children.

There was still not enough for Stalin. Sixteen years after Nadya's death, he arrested her close friend Polina Molotova, her sister Anna Redens, and her sister-in-law, Yevgenia Alliluyeva, because, he said, they "knew too much." Anna had committed the error of writing her memoirs, and although they were flattering to Stalin, he was still angry. She and Yevgenia were sentenced to ten years in prison. Anna's second husband was also arrested. Anna was released after Stalin died; she had, according to Svetlana, "gone mad in prison . . . having spent all six years of her imprisonment in solitary confinement, forbidden to correspond with her family, of whom she knew nothing during all that time."

Stalin also went after his other in-laws. He began the persecution of his first wife's family in 1937 with the arrest of her brother, A. S. Svanidze, along with Svanidze's wife Maria, their son, and Maria's sister and brother. The son was exiled to Kazakhstan, Svanidze was shot, and his wife and her sister died in prison. However, Svetlana attested that her father had loved the Svanidzes and "treated them like real members of the family."

This bizarre pattern was repeated over and over. No amount of friendship and loyalty was enough to win the dictator's trust. "The past ceased to exist for him," Svetlana observed. "Years of friendship and fighting side by side in a common cause might as well have never been. Difficult as it is to understand, he could wipe it all out in a stroke. . . . 'So you've betrayed me,' some inner demon would whisper. 'I don't even know you any more.' " The more people saw of Stalin, the better they knew him, the greater was their danger. Childhood friends, the valets who drank with him and procured women for him, the chiefs of the secret police who did his killing for him and knew everyone's scandals—all were killed. He was like a shark that mindlessly devours everything within reach of its jaws. Even when he had them helpless in prison, Stalin deceived his victims, promising to spare their lives and those of their families. He broke every promise.

SELF-IMPOSED HOUSE ARREST

Evidently, Stalin developed a fear of all human beings, and over the years he took unprecedented measures to protect himself from every imaginable danger. Lenin had been satisfied with two personal guards, whom he increased to four after an attempt was made on his life. Before 1933, according to Svetlana, her father followed Lenin's example: "The only guard was a man who rode in the car with my father and had nothing to do with the house. He wasn't allowed anywhere near it."

By 1937, the first year of the Great Purge, each of Stalin's residences was staffed and run by the secret police, and guards were everywhere. Eventually Stalin was guarded by several thousand men. The Kremlin, already a fortress, was strengthened and a second fortress was built underneath it, with tunnels exiting to strategic parts of Moscow. Stalin's houses were also fortified with underground chambers, perimeter walls, guard houses, searchlights, traps, and mines. The areas surrounding his homes were patrolled by detachments of soldiers with guard dogs. Khrushchev remarked: "Every time we got to the dacha [Stalin's Kuntsevo house], we used to whisper among ourselves about how there were more locks than the time before."

Visitors were searched, for no one was allowed in Stalin's presence carrying a weapon, although he always kept his own gun close by. He refused to eat or drink anything until someone else had tasted it first. Khrushchev made the accurate comment: "This shows that he had gone off the deep end. . . . He didn't trust anyone at all." Perhaps Stalin was particularly concerned about poison because he had ordered the liquidation of so many by that means. The dictator also had a laboratory for the testing of all his food and a doctor to test the air of his home at regular intervals.

Travel became vastly more complicated as Stalin grew more paranoid. When he made long trips by train, Stalin insisted that decoy trains precede his while security guards patrolled every foot of track over which he passed. For trips between the Kremlin and his home in Kuntsevo, he rode in an armored limousine with bullet-proof windows, curtains drawn, and a machine gun at the ready. There were always five cars in the cavalcade, all identical, which constantly changed order so that Stalin's could not be identified. All traffic was kept off the twelve-mile route, which was guarded by 3,000 agents.

Napoleon and Hitler, in their manic delusions that they were darlings of destiny, took few personal precautions against assassins. Although Hitler became increasingly inaccessible as defeat and depression destroyed his enthusiasm, he remained manically confident to the end. Not all manic depressives have the same delusions, however. Ironically, though Stalin lived longer than either Napoleon or Hitler, and was the only one of the three leaders who did not see his empire perish, he felt the least secure. His daughter attested: "At the peak of his glory and power he had experienced neither happiness nor satisfaction; instead, he was tormented by an eternal fear."

THE HIDDEN STALIN

The picture of Stalin's manic depression is incomplete. There are no accounts of marathon insomnia, no suicidal letters, no anecdotes about his hallucinations. Indeed, compared to what has been recorded about Napoleon and Hitler, there is little surviving information of any sort about the Georgian's inner life. Stalin immured himself behind a wall of silence. He died in power after a reign long enough for him to destroy most of the evidence about his personal affairs. He killed or imprisoned most of his family and friends, as well as anyone else who knew him well enough to have witnessed embarrassing moments and told about them. All those who remained near him and survived had to be taciturn and cautious. If Stalin had any confidants, either they kept his secrets or the secrets were buried with them. If they had any revealing letters from him, the letters were destroyed. Stalin censored his own past.

The tyrant presented himself to the world as the kindly, genial, all-knowing father of his country. Anyone who tried to tell a different story risked death. The information given here has come primarily from people who recorded their memories of the dictator after leaving the USSR. Khrushchev's memoirs had to be smuggled out of the country and published abroad.

However, for a quarter of a century, Stalin's mind and will were expressed both in the actions of the Soviety autocracy and in the lives of the Russian people. Although Stalin tried to project an idealized image of himself, so much of the truth has leaked out of the USSR over the years that what he actually was and did can be understood. Stalin was recognized in his own day as a "paranoiac." This was the clinical term used by a leading Soviet psychologist, Vladimir Bekhterev, who saw Stalin in 1927. Bekhterev also spoke of Stalin's grandiose delusions. Another who remarked on Stalin's "megalomania" and "sickly suspicion" was Khrushchev. Both these symptoms of psychosis are abundantly illustrated by Stalin's reign.

The most compelling evidence of Stalin's manic depression is to be found in the tyranny that was the political expression of his grandiose and paranoid delusions. This was evidence he could not suppress.

Part Five

A Brotherhood of Tyrants

16

Napoleon: Hitler's Ideal

As his life and career are studied, Napoleon emerges as a paradigm of the modern dictator, a forerunner of Hitler and Stalin. The resemblances are striking and unmistakable, both in small details and in overall patterns of behavior. Most striking of all are the parallels in their psychopathologies. All three men were afflicted with severe forms of manic depression in which grandiose and paranoid delusions made them utterly indifferent to human lives other than their own. These tyrants were champions of death.

THE DESPOTIC EGOTIST

A fundamental characteristic of all three tyrants was their dreadful egotism, a self-centeredness beyond the imagining of normal people. Napoleon could appear quite infantile in his self-regard. Throughout his life, he would instruct those around him, "Now, if I like somebody and honor him with my trust, I want to be the object of his dominant affection. I don't want to share, do you understand?" The corollary of this was jealousy of anyone who might offer competition. This vainglory made Napoleon—as it did Hitler and Stalin—easy prey for liars, toadies, and hypocrites. Napoleon rewarded only those who catered to his vanity: "Fools and scoundrels obtained from him decorations, titles, . . . and finally endowments," one witness noted, "which he refused or did not give to men of outstanding merit." Although Napoleon did not rid his government entirely of valuable people, his egocentricity had a stunting effect on those who remained. "Used as he was," his secretary attests, "to relate everything to himself, to see only himself, to admire only himself,

173

Napoleon paralyzed all about him. He wished for no glory but his own. He believed in no ability but his own."

Such a bloated ego does have some practical value for the tyrant. It urges him to praise himself without measure and persuades others to join him in the chorus of hosannas. Many people are apt to believe the praiseworthy things said about them, especially if all critical voices are silenced. "Through conceit, and especially through policy," a general said of Napoleon, "he lay claim to every achievement within the empire. . . . The rest of the world was long deluded by his advertising campaign, or deluded itself through . . . hero worship."

However, Bonaparte's relentless self-love and pursuit of "glory" eventually became intolerable burdens for the people who, forced to surrender their hard-won freedom and to sacrifice their loved ones to his ego, lived in the shadow of his power. A former supporter, the Vicomte de Chateaubriand, described the relief it was to have Napoleon gone: "We no longer see the conscription notices pasted up at street corners, and the passersby gathering in a crowd in front of those huge death-warrants, looking in consternation for the names of their children, their brothers, their friends . . . we forget that in the theater, the slightest remark directed against Bonaparte which had escaped the censor's notice was hailed with rapture. . . . Chateaubriand saw that Napoleon's ego had engulfed France. "Everything belonged to Bonaparte: '*I* have ordered, *I* have conquered, *I* have spoken; *my* eagles, *my* crown, *my* blood, *my* family, *my* subjects.' "

The tyrant's will acquires monstrous dimensions to match that of his ego, both making endless demands on anyone and everyone who might conceivably be able to obey the first and flatter the second. As in all Napoleon's relationships, whether with individuals or with the world, there was no equality. He refused to be constrained by anything himself, but expected to set the rules for everyone else, even deciding who would marry whom. Napoleon refused to play games honestly. When he lost a piece playing chess, he would sneak it back onto the board. He was indifferent to standards of dress even as emperor, he would go about with ink blotches on his clothing. "Civilization was always a little hateful to him," Talleyrand said of Napoleon.

Driven by impulse, the manic is frequently incapable of restraining his behavior in any way and becomes a law unto himself. Napoleon elevated this trait into a matter of principle, as he did with many of his manic characteristics. "I am not a man like other men: the laws of morality and decorum are not for me." Bonaparte was a political man without political principles, or principles of any other kind. Whatever could further his ambitions, he was willing to do. "There is only one thing to do in this world," Napoleon himself said, "and that is to keep acquiring more and more power. All the rest is chimerical." Napoleon's deadly grandiosity was unmistakable when he expressed his need to "assume universal dictatorship." To increase his power and protect what he had, he turned the Ministry of Police into a forerunner of the

Gestapo and the KGB. He ordered it to spy for him, to make arrests, and to kill on command, obedient to no law but his will. And to keep his guard dogs well-behaved, Napoleon had the Prefect of Police of Paris spy on the Ministry of Police, and vice versa, a method of control that Stalin would bring to perfection.

Napoleon also tried to impose thought-control on his subjects by confining art to propaganda and education to "directing political and moral opinion." Like Hitler and Stalin, Napoleon wanted to eliminate all loyalty except that to himself. He told the Gobelin tapestry makers to abandon the Bible as subject matter and substitute "the events that have created our throne." His attempts at thought control were not limited to instilling positive opinions about himself in the minds of his subjects:—he was determined to eliminate everything negative. Napoleon insisted, "Under my rule freedom of the press was unnecessary." He imprisoned people for publishing pamphlets that merely discussed the actions of his government. Critics of his policies and deeds were exiled. Compared to Hitler and Stalin, Napoleon's attempts at thought-control were primitive. However, he did not have their twentieth-century technology at his disposal.

In sum, Napoleon completely annulled the French Revolution. He restored the centralization of government, reimposed censorship, resumed the surveillance of citizens, and even recalled the aristocracy from exile to adorn his court. Neither defeats nor exile tempered his tyranny. His life demonstrated that manic dictators cannot be reformed—they must be removed.

DELUSIONS OF DIVINITY

Ultimately, the extremities of mania led Napoleon to believe that he had powers denied to the rest of humankind, that he was godlike—omnipotent, omniscient, and infallible. This is the sort of delusion that has immense potential for destruction. Napoleon wanted to impose his will on everything: "I have to look after the smallest details in person," he said. He expected everything to flow from his mind, from his orders, from his acts, as though from the hand of the Supreme Being.

Even early in his career, Bonaparte thought he was ready to join the ranks of Buddha, Christ, and Mohammed. "I was full of dreams," he said. "I saw myself founding a religion, marching into Asia, riding an elephant, a turban on my head and in my hand the new Koran that I would compose to suit my needs." While Napoleon never got around to writing a new Koran, he did have an imperial catechism distributed. "God has established him as our Sovereign," this strange document declared, "and has rendered him His image here on earth. . . . To honor and serve our Emperor is, therefore, to honor and serve God himself. . . . Those who fail in their duties toward our

Emperor, will render themselves deserving of eternal damnation." The Nazis would chant similar verses to Hitler while the Russians would maintain a cult of personality for Stalin.

Finally, the tyrant's feelings of omnipotence and omniscience grow as his political power becomes more absolute. Napoleon began his career with a relatively open mind. According to Chaptal, his first Minister of the Interior, "Bonaparte had one virtue which is more unusual the higher a man has risen. He was not ashamed of knowing so little of the details of general administration. He put many questions [and] incited discussion." Accordingly, "this period was marked by achievements . . . which have been admired by all Europe and will long be the pride of France." But during the interval 1800–1804 Napoleon's manic delusions took over, closing his mind to any information that could contradict or limit those delusions. At the same time, he removed from his government "all who had ability or character enough to be irksome," Chaptal continued. "He wanted flunkeys and not advisors, and had thus managed to isolate himself completely." On being contradicted, Napoleon often became violent, not caring whom he injured or what he destroyed. "When the Emperor asks for anyone's opinion, he expects it to be his own," said one companion. "You must never contradict him—never!" Merely to express insufficient enthusiasm about Napoleon's opinions or acts was to invoke frightful anger.

Blinded by his delusions, the manic tyrant refuses to believe that he has ever made any mistakes or is currently doing anything wrong. Napoleon would not believe in or even hear about the negative consequences of his own policies. When told about the hostility of the people his armies had for years plundered, raped, and injured, Napoleon was greatly astonished and hinted that his informant harbored treasonous sentiments. The delusional manic ignores warnings and rejects information that offends his ego. When Napoleon was brought bad news, he flew into a rage and the messenger was wise to keep out of sight for several days. People learned to avoid his explosions at all costs. A conspiracy of secrecy and pretense grew around him, reinforcing his delusions.

Had Napoleon been able to acknowledge his mistakes, he might have avoided repeating them, and would perhaps have settled for peace while he could still preserve some of his empire. But he was blinded by what a witness called his "unbounded trust in his arm and his genius." He was convinced that he could do no wrong but only great and wonderful things. Grandiose tyrants share this delusion. And since they fail to recognize the seriousness of a disaster they have caused, they often pile one calamity upon another.

Convinced of his omnipotence, Napoleon "never could see where the possible left off," one of his ministers noted. He eventually expected even nature to obey his will. One day Napoleon ordered his ships to leave the harbor so that he could inspect them at sea. On returning from a ride he saw that the ships had not moved. The admiral explained, "there is a frightful storm getting up. . . . Your Majesty does not wish to expose so many brave fellows to needless danger?" Infuriated, Napoleon banished the admiral to Holland and ordered the fleet out to sea. The storm sank many of Napoleon's ships, crashing them on the rocks. The drowning sailors' screams could be heard from the shore. Realizing that he had failed to control the weather and the ocean, Napoleon exclaimed, "Oh, the sea! It is revolting but I'll conquer it!"

THE CHAMPION OF DEATH

The most destructive delusion of the manic depressive tyrant is that all human lives but his own are expendable in the service of his glory and power. His willingness to sacrifice millions of lives in his pursuit of whatever he wants, be it territory, wealth, renown, adulation, victories, or some mirage of security, prepares him to become a champion of death.

Solitary arrogance is an incipient characteristic. Napoleon was both solitary and arrogant from his youth onward and became more inhuman as the years passed. While he expressed affection for people, he never reported having a sense of kinship with anyone. "The student of Brienne and the sublieutenant of artillery," General Caulaincourt recalled, "had acquaintances but no friends." This isolation became fundamental to Napoleon's character. Other people, Napoleon declared, "are as unlike myself as the moonlight is unlike the light of the sun." "Friendship is only an empty word," Napoleon said during his years of power. "I love nobody. No, I don't even love my brothers. . . . I know that I have no real friends."

Such isolation, egotism, and grandiosity eliminate all fellow feeling. This indifference to the amount and degree of suffering the manic depressive tyrant causes permits him to use the techniques of terror to enforce universal obedience. During his first campaign, Napoleon ordered Italian officials executed without trial and had entire towns burned to the ground with all their inhabitants slaughtered if one French soldier had been killed by a villager. That same pathological disregard of fellow human beings allowed Napoleon to send, without a qualm, huge numbers of his own soldiers to their deaths. Napoleon, his secretary noted, "regarded men as base coin, or as the tools with which he was to gratify his whims and ambitions. . . . While strolling across the battlefield of Eylau, on which 29,000 corpses lay, Napoleon shoved some of the bodies with his foot, remarking to the generals who accompanied him: " 'Small change.' "

Believing that he is greater than all of humanity, the champion of death will choose to eliminate mankind if he faces the loss of his power. Like Hitler at the imminent defeat of Germany, Napoleon was prepared to destroy the world. He promised that if he lost his throne, "I will bury the world beneath its ruins!" In time, virtually all the people of Europe came to realize what a monster Napoleon was—except perhaps the French. But one of his countrymen, Chateaubriand, observed, "In his lifetime Napoleon was regarded as the devil let loose upon Europe. His character, his explosiveness and incalculability, his boundless determination to impose his will, produced in his enemies a mystical sense of horror."

17

Hitler: A Champion of Death

TYRANNY AND MADNESS

With respect to some of its effects on character and behavior, severe mania can be viewed as a disorder of will and identity. The will of the manic wants to control everything and does not tolerate frustrations or disappointments well. In the most extreme stages of mania, the will becomes inflated with grandiose fantasies; some sufferers develop delusions that they have divine powers, that whatever they want must come to be. The manic identity displays its first distortions by an exaggerated self-esteem, which may become, in the psychotic stages, delusions that the manic speaks for God, is an agent of God with divinely ordained missions, or has become a god himself.

As such unstable tyrants progress toward their delusory divinity, they demand increasing adulation and power, with the appetite of an addiction that grows the more it is fed. As they retreat into delusion, they become increasingly dangerous. Unfortunately, while they grow less and less rational, they pursue power with greater ferocity. It is a vicious circle: power feeding delusion, which increases the hunger for more power. Hitler's press officer, Otto Dietrich, observed, "as his power grew, his arbitrariness became more and more absolute." Dietrich also saw that "Hitler's imagination unconsciously created a vast delusional world in order to give his egotism room to hold sway."

Only a particular type of manic depressive develops delusions of divinity, and only a small minority of manic depressives possess the qualifications to succeed in political careers. The dangerous individual is he who belongs to both groups, for he is the stuff of which tyrants are made. The brotherhood of tyrants—Napoleon, Hitler, and Stalin—as they developed their delusions of divinity while exercising absolute power, behaved in startlingly similar ways —and this despite the great differences in their personal histories, talents, and educations as well as the dissimilarities in the cultures, histories, and economies of the nations they ruled, and the disparate routes to power that they took. What the three had in common were the mania and paranoia that in their psychotic intensity gave rise to monstrous dreams.

THE DESPOTIC SOLIPSIST

The manic depressive tyrant, in the darkest corners of his twisted logic, is as alone in the world as a solipsist, for he does not acknowledge that anyone else has a right to exist. Those who live in proximity to someone aspiring to omnipotence become the tyrant's possessions, with no more freedom than if they were articles of clothing. Press chief Dietrich recorded that no one who belonged to Hitler "could resign without his permission." However, being the tyrant's property does not provide any security, for it implies no obligation on the part of the tyrant to take care of the person he owns. Even those who were perfectly loyal and submissive to Hitler for many years were suddenly demoted or dismissed during his rages.

Not only is the tyrant the sole significant human being in his mental universe, his is the only will. Speaking to the Nazi party, Hitler said: "Nothing happens in this movement except what I wish." The führer's need to feel all-powerful also affected how his government operated. Dietrich reported that "his impulse to dominate was a consuming fire. . . . Decisions were . . . passed on to the government and the party as accomplished facts. . . . Anyone who did not obey his orders without question was branded a defeatist and a saboteur." Those who did not obey at all fared worse. "Whoever fails to obey my orders," Hitler declared, "will be destroyed. I shall strike as soon as I have so much as a suspicion of their disobedience."

Of course, the tyrant's obsession with power is, in the long run, self-defeating. People who do not share the tyrant's belief in his divine prerogatives resent his crushing of their personalities, as one of Hitler's aides testified: "Those working in close association with Hitler were constantly torn between admiration, . . . despair, disappointment and hatred." By imposing his will without limit, the tyrant turns loyal followers into disguised enemies, thus undermining his own power, and this is a process that may end by destroying him, for he is nothing without followers.

Like Stalin and Napoleon, Hitler interfered with every aspect of his subjects' lives. The führer dictated statutes that decreed the religion of household servants, he ruled on the colors which artists could use in their paintings, he determined how physics was taught in universities. He decided whom Germans could marry, what they could name their children, and where they could be buried. The only time the German people had any respite from Hitler's meddling was when he was too depressed to think of new laws.

All three dictators in our study were determined to eliminate whatever could challenge or limit their power. Hitler could have been paraphrasing Napoleon's statements when he said: "Never suffer the rise of two continental powers in Europe. Regard any attempt to organize a second military power on the German frontiers, even if only in the form of creating a state capable of military strength, as an attack on Germany." If any such state arose, he continued, "smash it." Using the excuse over and over that he made war only to prevent other countries from attacking Germany, Hitler assembled an empire even more extensive than that of Napoleon. The largest empire of all time belonged to Stalin, who merely wanted all the territory bordering what he had and also whatever was on the borders of the new acquisitions, ad infinitum.

THE DELUSION OF OMNISCIENCE

From adolescence, Hitler believed himself a genius, which he defined as having innate knowledge. In actuality, he never displayed any intellectual prowess except for an excellent memory. "I often ask myself," he said, "how one human brain could preserve so many facts." The facts were limited to armaments and architecture. In addition, Hitler notably lacked intellectual curiosity and avoided whatever might challenge his preconceptions. As Dietrich reported, "Hitler certainly had innumerable opportunities for conversation with important and interesting people [but he] . . . never made use of these opportunities. . . . He remained perpetually in the same company . . . in the same stage of monotony and boredom, producing eternally the same speeches and declarations." Though Hitler read some biography and history, he never allowed what he read to penetrate his delusions about the Aryans, the Jews, and the destiny of Germany. In his first years as chancellor, Hitler reread his favorite boyhood fare, the fantasies about the American West concocted by Karl May.

All the communications media in Germany became tools that Hitler used to stamp belief in his genius on the minds of the public. The press he controlled called him "an unassailable expert. . . . Nobody will be able to measure his great depth." The führer was also "the highest synthesis of the race," and embodied "the universalism of Goethe, the depth of Kant, the dynamism of Hegel, the . . . genius of Frederic II, . . . the tumultuous inspiration of Wagner."

Not only was Hitler omniscient, his manic grandiosity assured him that no one but he knew anything. He was referring to himself when he said, "The creative genius stands always outside the circle of experts." In order for Hitler to accept an idea, he had to think it originated with him. "There was no way of influencing that will of his," Dietrich noted, adding that Hitler made important decisions "by himself . . . and considered them as intuitive inspiration." While Napoleon developed a closed mind, Hitler's began that way. "He was unteachable," Dietrich said. "With unparalleled intellectual arrogance and biting irony he dismissed anything that did not fit with his own ideas."

Moreover, Hitler had little use for the veneer of civilization, declaring that he wanted Germany's youth to be "violently active, dominating, intrepid, brutal. . . . I want to see once more in its eyes the gleam of pride and independence of the beast of prey. . . . I shall eradicate the thousands of years of human domestication. . . . I will have no intellectual training." Lacking any real formal training himself, the führer demanded intellectual as well as moral regression: "Providence has ordained that I should be the greatest liberator of humanity. I am freeing men from the restraints of an intelligence that has taken charge; from the dirty and degrading self-mortification of a chimera called conscience and morality." In effect, Hitler preached a gospel of criminality. "We are ruthless. I have no bourgeois scruples! . . . Yes, we are barbarians!" That was part of Hitler's appeal, and it is one of the secrets of many a demagogue's allure.

THE DELUSION OF INFALLIBILITY

Hitler declared, "I hereby set forth for myself and my successors in the leadership of the party the claim of political infallibility. I hope the world will grow accustomed to that claim as it has to the claim of the Holy Father." But he was not limiting his claim to politics: "I never make a mistake," Hitler declared categorically.

When the disastrous outcome of the führer's plans threatened his claim to infallibility, he either blamed others or resorted to paranoia. "He always preferred," Dietrich said, "to hide his own defeats by charging sabotage." In 1932, Hitler had exclaimed "I want war." He also insisted, "Without power over Europe we must perish." But he did not win the war, so in his last will, thirteen years later, Hitler blamed the war on the Jews, saying that the conflict was "provoked exclusively by those international statesmen who were of Jewish origin or worked for Jewish interests."

THE DELUSION OF OMNIPOTENCE

The manic tyrant demonstrates his belief in the infinity of his power by inaugurating gargantuan projects, regardless of their cost and relevancy to the needs of his subjects. Hitler planned for the Nazi party headquarters in Nuremberg to have outer walls 270 feet high, using six million bricks for the foundations alone. Forty miles of new railroad track would have been needed just to permit the excavations to be dug. He wanted to erect the largest building in the world, the design for which came to him while writing *Mein Kampf* in prison.

Hitler also decided to annex the United States to Germany and turn it into a German-speaking nation. Giving no thought to the difficulties involved, he argued: "America is permanently on the brink of revolution. It will be a simple matter for me to produce unrest and revolts in the United States." Albert Speer commented on Hitler's ambitions: "[A]ll his endeavors were from the beginning limitless and irrational. That holds true for architecture; it holds true for the war, which was planned long in advance, and likewise for the economic program, the dictatorship, and finally the annihilation of human beings." Napoleon had merely wanted to equal the career of Alexander the Great. The führer aspired to considerably more—the remodeling of the human race. "Those who see in National Socialism nothing more than a political movement," Hitler said, "know scarcely anything of it. . . . [I]t is the will to create mankind anew."

WORSHIPING HITLER

Like Napoleon, the führer had a yearning to be worshiped by foreigners: "I'm going to become a religious figure," he announced. "Soon I'll be the great chief of the Tartars. Already Arabs and Moroccans are mingling my name with their prayers." Stalin's pathology in this regard was close to Hitler's: they both required such adulation that "cults of personality" developed around them to meet their needs. These cults were the crystallization of three themes: that the dictators were kindly, loving fathers of their people; that they were universal geniuses; and that they were divine. Many political leaders incorporate kindly fatherhood into their political personae. It is in the worship of an autocratic leader's putative genius and divinity that public relations are metamorphosed into the absurd and frightening irrationalities of the dictator's cult, and the mind-slavery of the totalitarian state appears in the measures used to promote the cult.

The cult's image of the dictator becomes as delusional as the thinking of the man it celebrates. One officially sanctioned treatise described Hitler as "a pure Aryan type" with blond hair. The function of the cult is to substitute its fantasies for reality in the minds of the dictator's subjects so that they think, feel, and act as the dictator desires. Hitler, however, left nothing to chance: Germany's Academy of Law was directed to proclaim that one was legally bound to love the führer, and dislike of him was therefore criminal.

Initially his followers exalted Germany above Hitler: "He who serves Adolf Hitler serves Germany, and he who serves Germany serves God," said the head of the Hitler Youth. But soon Hitler evolved into an agent of God. "We need no priests or parsons," his followers said. "We communicate directly with God through Adolf Hitler." People were expected to pray: "Führer, my führer, sent to me from God, protect and maintain me throughout my life. Thou who hast saved Germany from deepest need, I thank thee today for my daily bread. Remain at my side and never leave me, führer, my führer, my faith, my light."

But even that was not enough—Hitler had to become God's equal. The Minister for Justice declared, "Hitler is lonely. So is God. Hitler is like God." Special prayers were written for the children of Germany: "As Jesus freed men from sin and Hell, so Hitler freed the German people from destruction. Jesus and Hitler were persecuted, but while Jesus was crucified, Hitler was raised to the chancellorship. . . . Jesus strove for heaven, Hitler for the German earth."

Clearly, Hitler had won the competition. The leader of the Nazi party in the Saar region proclaimed "Hitler is a new, a greater, and more powerful Jesus Christ." Germans were told: "Adolf is the real Holy Ghost" and "Hitler's word is God's law, the decrees and laws which represent it possess divine authority." The young had to pledge: "I consecrate my life to Hitler; I am ready to die for Hitler, my savior." Other prayers were directed to Hitler as God Himself: "Adolf Hitler, you are our great Leader. Thy name makes the earth tremble. Thy Third Reich comes, thy will alone is law upon earth. Let us hear daily thy voice and order us by thy leadership, for we will obey to the end even with our lives." These prayers were the answer to a grandiose manic's most fervent wish: every fantasy, every demand of will and ego were met.

This religion was made part of national policy by government decree, which established the National Reich Church of Germany to incorporate and control all of the churches in Hitler's empire. The new church declared that "the greatest written document of our people is the book of our führer, *Mein Kampf.* It is completely aware that this book incorporates not only the greatest, but also the purest and truest ethics for the present life of our people." Every congregation had to empty its altars of all crucifixes, Bibles, and pictures of saints, replacing them with copies of *Mein Kampf.* The swastika would substitute for crosses on all churches. Hitler took his divinity seriously, informing an audience in 1933 that if he failed to become "the power and the glory," and to bring Germany into a new kingdom, "You should crucify me." However, he did not insist upon it when the occasion arose.

The führer eventually announced that he had reached a "superhuman state," having become "more godlike than human." Hitler also declared that his godlike condition placed him "above the law," where he was "bound by none of the conventions of human morality."

BLUEPRINT FOR A CHAMPION OF DEATH

The limitless ego-expansion of the absolute ruler is the most dangerous aspect of his character, for the tyrant comes to value himself above all humanity, which he considers a separate and inferior species. The process first becomes noticeable as the leader limits his contact with others. Speer observed, "his style of rule led Hitler, especially after 1937, into increasing isolation. Added to that was his inability to make human contacts." Speer added, "The genial, relaxed Hitler whom I had known in the early '30s had become, even to his intimate entourage, a forbidding despot with few human relationships."

As time went on, the führer also reduced his contact with the German people, and instead of going out among them watched movies every night. Consequently, he derived from his propaganda-serving film industry rather glamorous notions of what was happening in his country. Finally, Hitler gave up even this shadowy version of reality. The only film that he saw thereafter was *Napoleon Is to Blame for Everything.*

The more godlike Hitler seemed to himself, the more contempt he felt for others. The führer stated: "Extraordinary geniuses permit of no consideration for normal mankind." He was contemptuous of his power base, the Germans, calling them "as stupid as they are forgetful," "weak and bestial," "crazy and cowardly," and "the great stupid mutton herd of our sheeplike people." Hitler declared: "If you wish the sympathy of the broad masses, then you must tell them the crudest and most stupid things"—which is exactly what he did. Although they had chosen him, Hitler considered the Germans incapable of selecting a good leader. "The revulsion of the masses for outstanding genius is positively instructive." After his election Hitler said, "What luck for governments that the peoples they administer don't think. . . . If it were otherwise, the state of society would be impossible." He declared that the best way to assure having a good breed of Germans was to kill seventy to eighty percent of all German babies born each year, saving only the best.

The inevitable corollary of these crazed notions was that other lives do not matter in the least. Like Napoleon, Stalin, and many other tyrants, Hitler's ego metastasized to the point that he felt his country existed only for his benefit. One of his top generals, Franz Halder, attested that "there was for him no Germany, there were no German troops for whom he felt responsible; for him there was . . . only one greatness, a greatness which dominated his life and to which his evil genius sacrificed everything—his own Ego." One of Hitler's aides recalled that those "in führer's headquarters found reason to hate him for his acts of ruthlessness, hardness, injustice, and brutality . . . as for instance . . . when he directed the ruthless sacrifice of . . . whole divisions."

The führer left no doubt that he was prepared to sacrifice all of Germany to his own ego: "I shall become the greatest man in history," he promised. "I have to gain immortality even if the whole German nation perishes in the process." By 1939 Hitler was even contemplating the sacrifice of all humanity on the altar of his self-esteem. He said: "We shall not capitulate—no, never. We may be destroyed, but if we are, we shall drag a world with us—a world in flames." Then he hummed a theme from Wagner's apocalytpic vision, the *Götterdämmerung*.

HATRED AND VENGEANCE

Hitler and Stalin were both filled with deep-seated hatreds and their power enabled them to express these hatreds in genocidal policies. The only difference was that the German dictator, having imposed his own twisted religion and ethics on his people, had no need for hypocrisy. He said that God's "most beautiful gift to us is the hatred of our enemies, whom we in turn hate with all our hearts." The one stable element amidst the violent zigzags of Hitler's moods was hatred, which amounted almost to an obsession. Dr. Rauschning noted, "Every conversation, however unimportant, seemed to show that this man was filled with an immeasurable hatred. . . . Almost anything might suddenly inflame his wrath and his hatred." Hatred also seeped into Hitler's private relationships. Speer reported that the führer "seemed to enjoy destroying the reputation and self-respect of even his closest associates and faithful comrades."

Hitler's hatred was not confined to those near at hand and those who hated him directly. When the German armies invaded Poland in 1939, Hitler ordered the extermination of the Polish gentry, the Polish intelligentsia, and much of the clergy as well as Poland's Jews. The sight of Warsaw bombed and burning inspired him to exclaim, "That is how we will annihilate them." Of the six million Poles who were killed, less than one million were battlefield casualties. The work of the SS extermination gangs that followed the German armies into Russia was even more appalling, and this despite the fact that many Russians welcomed the Germans as liberators from Stalin.

Hitler instituted slave labor, which often was equivalent to execution. Laborers were routinely beaten to death or died of cold, untreated illness, or starvation. The penalty for "loafing" or any refusal to work was hanging. Wherever the Germans invaded, people were kidnaped and families separated. Entire towns were kidnaped, too, and their houses burned to the ground, to provide slave labor for the industries of the Reich.

Toward the end of the war, Hitler dragged as many people to death with him as he could. He needlessly insisted, as his troops left the city, on the destruction of Paris. He ordered all prisoners of war killed. Although Germans fleeing from advancing Russian armies were using them as shelter, Hitler ordered the tunnels leading into Berlin flooded. He sent adolescent boys to make suicidal attacks against the Soviet troops. Press secretary Otto Dietrich recognized that Hitler was taking vengeance against the German people. "He asked the impossible of them, and when they did not meet his standards he said they had no right to life." Hitler ultimately blamed his defeat on the German people. "Germany is not worthy of me; let her perish."

The total number of those who died because of Hitler's mad ambitions and hatreds has been counted and recounted many times during the last half century. To the millions who fell in the battles of his senseless war must be added many millions more who perished in prisoner of war and concentration camps or in the savage pogroms of the SS. Yet other millions died of starvation and disease caused by the war's dislocations. And the world has continued to suffer from numerous smaller wars caused by the turmoils Hitler's huge conflict left behind. Humankind has paid a dreadful price for not recognizing that it was dealing with a paranoid, manic depressive megalomaniac whose illness made him capable of the most monstrous crimes—indeed, made him eager to commit them. It was not for lack of warning. Through the 1920s, before he came to power, Hitler loudly advertised what he intended to do once he ruled Germany. In 1939, shortly before he started the war, he summed up his terrible purposes. "Do I intend to eradicate whole races? Of course I do." If he had been taken seriously, he could have been stopped then.

18

Stalin: The Enemy of the People

CANCEROUS EGO

Manic tyrants labor under the rule of a despotic ego compelling them to devote their existence to nothing but what promotes their power and increases their conceit, even to sacrifice their nations in the defense of their self-esteem. Tremendous vanity, envy, and susceptibility to adulation are the hallmarks of this obsession with self.

An uncommon taste for flattery, common in manics, becomes an insatiable appetite in the tyrant. Stalin's hunger for praise was evident as early as the 1920s. A friend of that time complained, "I am doing everything he has asked me to do, but it is still not enough for him. He wants me to admit he is a genius." Even when he had gained enormous power, Stalin continued to demand adulation. Lavrenti Beria, perhaps the most hard-boiled of Stalin's secret police chiefs, learned that fawning was the way to his master's heart. "He flattered my father with a shamelessness that was nothing if not Oriental," recalled Stalin's daughter Svetlana. "He praised him and made up to him in a way that caused old friends . . . to wince with embarrassment."

The other side of this was Stalin's consuming jealousy, a symptom of depression. He could not bear for anyone else to receive praise. He was driven, Trotsky stated, by "an active, never slumbering envy of all who are more gifted, more powerful, rank higher than he." Another Bolshevik leader, Nikolai Bukharin, observed, "If anybody speaks better than Stalin, his doom is sealed. . . . Such a man is a constant reminder to him that he is not the first, the best. If anybody writes better, so much the worse for him because *he*, Stalin, only he should be the first Russian writer."

The unrelenting selfishness of many manics was also prominent in Stalin's personality. One seeks in vain for instances that showed his concern for others. Except for a few recorded instances of tenderness for his daughter, Svetlana, Stalin was uninhibited by consideration for his children and made no effort to compensate them for the loss of their mother. "Stalin always went on holidays alone," Khrushchev noted. "He never took his children with him." Svetlana was Stalin's favorite but, according to Khrushchev, as she grew older, "he never showed any parental tenderness. When he wasn't being downright abusive toward her, he was cold and unfeeling."

Like Hitler, Napoleon, and many other tyrannical manic types, Stalin's life was dedicated solely to his own power and glory. Trotsky observed, "In each new situation his first and foremost consideration was how he personally could benefit. Whenever the interests of the whole came into conflict with his personal interests, he always without exception sacrificed the interests of the whole."

THE DISEASED WILL

The manic tyrant is satisfied with nothing less than total control over all others, but he accepts no restraints to his own will and disregards rules and laws of any kind that might interfere with his desires. Stalin's daughter noted: "There lay in him a firm conviction that the precept about using any means to attain an end produced far greater results than lofty ideals ever could." In the Soviet Union under Stalin's rule, hypocrisy replaced ethics and law was whatever he said it was.

Tyranny usually begins at home, as it did where Stalin resided. His daughter attested: "He wanted no equals . . . he wanted blind devotion and absolute submission to his will." Perfect obedience was not enough. Stalin wanted to plant all the thoughts in everyone's head. Svetlana observed: "In everyone he wanted to find lowered eyes and silent acquiescence. He could not tolerate a personal opinion in others." Or any personal desires. When Svetlana told her father that she wanted to marry, he said, "So you want to get married, do you? To hell with you."

Taking measure of his leader, Khrushchev said that Stalin "had a bully's personality." At the last New Year's Eve party Stalin gave before his death, he and his colleagues sang and danced to Russian and Georgian folk music being played on a phonograph. When Svetlana arrived her father insisted that she join in the dancing, though she was visibly tired. She obeyed, but soon stopped, leaning exhausted against a wall. Stalin insisted "You're the hostess, so dance!" She replied "I've already danced, Papa, I'm tired." Khrushchev relates, "With that, Stalin grabbed her by the forelock of her hair and pulled. I could see her face turning red and tears welling up in her eyes. He pulled harder and dragged her back onto the dance floor."

While Stalin subjected those he considered enemies to a life of slavery in his camps, his political cronies endured a slavery of a more intimate nature. A high Soviet official noted: "Stalin does not need advisors, he needs only executors . . . he demands from his closest aides complete submission, obedience, subjection—unprotesting, slavish discipline."

Stalin completed the subjugation of his associates by involving them in his crimes. Voroshilov, who was placed at the head of the army, was during the great Purge made an accomplice to the destruction of his military friends and colleagues. Mikhail Kalinin, the Soviet President, was told to sign the death sentences of his closest friends. He obeyed, weeping. Despite Kalinin's cooperation, his wife was imprisoned in 1937 and tortured. After the war, when Stalin's old and faithful colleague Molotov had the temerity to abstain from voting for his own wife's exile, Stalin went into a rage and, reported Khrushchev, "started kicking Molotov around viciously."

The tyrant's will lay over his nation like a glacier, freezing, smothering, crushing, and pulverizing everything beneath it. By 1940 virtually all aspects of Russian life were supervised by organizations that took their orders directly from Stalin. He oversaw and meddled in every sort of enterprise: agriculture, manufacturing transportation, commerce, education, science, the arts, medical services, the news media, internal and external travel, and housing. He set prices and wages and dictated the people's social activity He made his people sing hymns to his Five-Year Plans. He rewarded them for having large families. Foreign observers during the war were astonished to see Stalin meddling in everything: diplomacy, protocol, strategy, tactics, and army supplies. Taking manic domination to the ultimate degree, Stalin insisted on making the most detailed decisions himself.

THE IMAGINARY STALIN

"Paper will put up with anything that is written on it," Stalin once observed, and the *Short Biography* that he had published in 1948 proved it. The work was filled with "examples of loathsome adulation," Khrushchev said. Moreover, the lies "were approved and edited by Stalin personally and some of them were added in his own handwriting. . . . He marked the very places where he thought that the praises of his services were insufficient." With a strain of mock-modesty, the Georgian made sure to insert: "Stalin never allowed his work to be marred by the slightest hint of vanity, conceit, or self-adulation."

Rarely was Stalin sincere except when expressing his anger and paranoia. Virtually everything else was pretense designed to create the impression that he was moderate and benevolent. But at the center of each performance was the core of Stalin's own delusions. The dictator cherished a manic faith in the fantastic image he presented to the world, just as he came to believe the propaganda movies generated by the Soviet film industry. One of Stalin's favorite fantasies was that he was another Napoleon. Not satisfied merely with awarding medals to himself, he insisted on managing, or rather, mismanaging his country's armed forces.

Stalin tried to infect others with his grandiose delusion that he was a brave and brilliant military leader. In August of 1943, he put off meeting with Roosevelt and Churchill on the grounds that "I have frequently to go to different sectors of the front," and "I had not the opportunity to leave the front for even one week." That month Stalin had himself photographed at a place which had been prepared to look like a front-line command post, and he plastered the country with posters and paintings of himself at the front: that was as close to the fighting as he ever went. One of Stalin's generals attested, "not once did his eyes behold a soldier in combat."

The version of the war that Stalin created was a thoroughgoing fantasy glorifying both him and the USSR. He told military historians that there had been no defeats because he had planned all along to draw the German forces deep into Russia in order to destroy them. After the war, Stalin's generals gave him credit for his organizational ability, which was charitable of them, although he gave them credit for nothing. When some of his commanders took actions contrary to his orders, he claimed responsibility for the resulting victories. According to Khrushchev, "Stalin excluded every possibility that services rendered at the front should be credited to anyone but himself." The dictator had official propaganda denigrate the military leaders and heroes who had actually won the war, while publicizing himself as the person solely responsible for victory.

In part, he was motivated by fear that the generals' prestige would make them too popular for his own security, and after the war he again entrusted the most important military commands only to relative nonentities. But the propaganda campaign was also motivated by Stalin's tyrannical ego. He inserted into his official biography statements such as: "At the various stages of the war Stalin's genius found the correct solutions that took account of all the circumstances of the situation." He had the biography describe him as "the sublime strategist of all times and nations." Though he had insisted on the manufacture of obsolete weapons, Stalin added: "The advanced Soviet science of war received further development at Comrade Stalin's hands."

THE SOVIET ICON

Stalin's insatiable demand for praise "gave birth," Khrushchev noted, "to many flatterers and specialists in false optimism and deceit." One of the most unctuous of Stalin's admirers could hardly contain himself. "Every time I have found myself in his presence I have been subdued by his strength, his charm, his grandeur. I have experienced a great desire to sing, to cry out, to shout with joy and happiness." Another enthusiast rejoiced in Stalin's name, "which is strong, beautiful, wise and marvelous. Thy name is engraven on every factory, every machine, every place on earth."

Images of Stalin—excluding his pockmarks and all signs of aging—were mass-produced. An American general observed in 1950 that "the people are seldom out of sight of his statue or his picture" The Man of Steel became the icon of his nation. Soviet writer Ilya Ehrenberg stated: "In the minds of millions Stalin was transformed into a mythical demigod: everyone trembled as they said his name, [and] believed that he alone could save the Soviet Union from invasion and collapse." "The cult of the individual," Khrushchev said, "acquired such monstrous size chiefly because Stalin himself, using all conceivable methods, supported the glorification of his own person." The cult was so effective that after his death and the subsequent revelations about his crimes, many Russians—perhaps the majority—were still unable to surrender their faith in his benevolence and greatness.

THE OMNISCIENT COMRADE

The first to believe in his mythical qualities was the dictator himself. While Stalin never developed the manic delusion that he was invulnerable, he did come to see himself as the possessor of divine attributes: omniscience, infallibility and omnipotence.

Stalin behaved as though he were omniscient when drawing up the first Five-Year Plan. He ignored the data collected by economists and government officials; thenceforward, the Five-Year Plans were based on what he wanted done rather than on the information available. In his grandiosity Stalin did not trouble to investigate actual conditions, and punished those who tried to intrude truth into his delusions. The Director of the Institute of Economics of the USSR Academy of Sciences was killed for informing Stalin during the war that the United States still surpassed the USSR in agriculture and labor productivity.

Stalin's grandiose delusions and willful ignorance continued to hamper the Soviet economy after the war. He retarded the development of the chemical industry by deciding that oil and gas, despite the Soviet Union's huge and valuable reserves, were unimportant. Agriculture, which was still struggling to recover from the effects of the war, was further burdened with additional taxes. Any experts who disagreed with his plans were accused of defeatism and risked imprisonment as traitors. Those who survived simply told Stalin what he wanted to hear. The inflated reports needed to satisfy Stalin's grandiose demands became part of the political and military tradition of the Soviet Union.

Stalin had the politician's memory for names and faces, and like Hitler he remembered specifications of weapons. He also remembered those aspects of industrial technology that interested him. Like Napoleon, Stalin attended to details and work diligently, at least until the post-war years. But none of this qualified him to tell geologists where oil was to be found, nor did it make him competent to advise physicians about their specialties, biologists about genetics and physicists about atomic theory.

As early as 1929, when he was fifty, Stalin had become convinced that he was a universal expert. The dictator could no longer distinguish between his ideas and the laws of nature, between his desires and the way nations develop. His became not only the final word on science, philosophy and all the arts but the only word. Reality, in effect, was no more and no less than what he said it was at any given moment as he insisted that the Communist world adopt his psychotic worldview.

Stalin finally claimed to possess an ability akin to mind-reading or clair-voyance. "Comrade Stalin's genius enabled him to divine the enemy's plans and defeat them," the *Short Biography* claimed. Stalin also became convinced of his infallibility: "He is after all a 'genius,' and a genius cannot help but be right," wrote Khrushchev sardonically. "Everyone can err, but Stalin considered that he never erred, that he was always right. He never acknowledged that he made any mistake, large or small." Stalin also behaved as though his conduct were perfect: "Apologies were alien to his very nature," Khrushchev observed. Napoleon's and Hitler's egos were equally unbending—and equally intolerant of the existence of independent thinking. Says Khrushchev: "Stalin could not stand to have his ideas questioned or deliberated. He might let you talk to him if you agreed with him. Sometimes he told you to shut up no matter what you were saying." On one occasion the dictator denied that Holland was a member of Benelux (an economic union between Belgium, the Netherlands, and Luxembourg). When the Yugoslav Foreign Minister tried to correct him, Stalin replied angrily: "When I say no it means no!" One Soviet strategist who summoned the nerve to contradict Stalin's military doctrines was imprisoned and not released until after the dictator's death.

Disagreement with Stalin could be fatal. "Stalin originated the concept 'enemy of the people,' " noted Khrushchev, adding that "this term made possible the usage of the most cruel repression, violating all norms of revolutionary legality, against anyone who in any way disagreed with Stalin." When Nikolai Voznesensky, whom Stalin had installed in the Politburo, suggested that the economy would benefit from less centralized planning, Stalin accused him of trying to return the USSR to capitalism and had him shot immediately.

The dictator maintained a facade of perfection and infallibility by pinning his defects on others. He accused people of wearing "masks," of "putting the interests of [one's] ego higher than those of truth," of conceit and megalomania, and of "laying one's own fault at another's door."

DELUSIONS OF OMNIPOTENCE

In 1949 Stalin announced a "Plan For the Transformation of Nature" that, through irrigation and reforestation, would make the USSR an agricultural wonder. He elevated the harebrained genetic theories of Trofim Lysenko to the status of Holy Writ because they stated that plants and animals could be made into almost anything Stalin desired through the inheritance of changes that took place during growth. Lysenko promised that he could change wheat into rye and make valuable crops flourish where neither soil nor climate were hospitable. Stalin damned Mendelian genetics as heretical. Any scientist who expressed disagreement with Stalin's outrageous views was accused of everything from racism to sabotage to being an agent of imperialist capitalism. If he did not recant he lost his laboratory, his employment and sometimes his freedom—such as it was. Stalin also came to believe that the ideas inculcated by relentless propaganda would be inherited down the generations. Thus the tyrant would become the ultimate creator of Soviet man.

CONTINENTAL DELUSIONS

Stalin applied his grandiose delusions about himself to his country. Since he was the only genius in the USSR, his country had to be the only source of genius in the world. After 1949, it was declared that the Russians, not Guttenberg, were the original inventors of the printing press and that such modern inventions as the telegraph, telephone, radio, bicycle, tractor, tank, airplane, and rocket were entirely Russian creations. The Russians, according to his view, were an omniscient nation.

Stalin insisted that everyone agree that—with a few trivial exceptions—the Soviet Union was a veritable Utopia filled with prosperous, contented people who worked enthusiastically, were enchanted with communism, and stood united behind their leader. Beyond that, Stalin's delusions demanded that his fellow citizens reflect his infallibility and never make mistakes, nor have personal failings, nor incur accidents.

Artists, historians, journalists, and scientists were compelled to express this dream of Russian perfection or else have their work and careers destroyed, and risk their lives as well. Willing or not, they became his accomplices in fantasy. Thus completing the circle of delusion, Stalin relied on these producers of dreams-on-demand for information about what was happening in the Soviet Union.

In Stalin's perfect Russia, tick infestations were the work of saboteurs, as were harvests that failed to meet expectations. All fires became arson. The poor quality of goods and shortages resulted from the ingenuity of enemy agents. Accidents caused by worn-out equipment or administrative oversight were also classified as sabotage, and the "saboteurs" were killed. In Stalin's Soviet heaven, everyone agreed with him; therefore only one candidate, approved by the dictator, was presented for each electoral office. People could vote "no," but their votes were not counted. For Stalin, "no" did not exist, unless *he* said it.

A PENITENTIARY CALLED RUSSIA

Xenophobia, an outgrowth of his paranoia, invaded not only the dictator's life, but touched, and sometimes shortened, the lives of his fellow citizens. He decreed that none of them could marry anyone from another country. The law was repealed soon after Stalin's death, but a law barring Soviet citizens from "furnishing information," including street directions, to a foreigner was still in effect twenty years later. Stalin reacted to objects originating outside of Russia as though they were sources of infection. His daughter recalled, "To the end of his days my father would ask me with a look of real displeasure, 'Is that something foreign you've got there?' " Xenophobia was an unadmitted but powerful factor in Stalin's foreign policy. In 1952, foreign diplomats were denied access to all but twenty of the USSR's cities and towns. The Indian Embassy was forced to relocate because it was on Stalin's route from his Kuntsevo home to the Kremlin, and the American Embassy had to move because the Kremlin was visible from its location. Most of the leaders of neutral, nonaligned countries, which often appeared to American observers as leftist, were denounced by Stalin as "imperialist agents."

Delusional suspicions and fears prompted Stalin to make the USSR a garrison state. Khrushchev admitted: "He overemphasized the importance of military might, for one thing, and consequently put too much faith in our armed forces. He lived in terror of an enemy attack. For him foreign policy meant keeping the anti-aircraft unit around Moscow on a twenty-four-hour alert."

THE MIND OF THE GENOCIDE

As we have already observed in the cases of Napoleon and Hitler, the fundamental difference between ordinary people and the tyrant who sacrifices millions of lives is that the tyrant feels no kinship with, no enduring connection to, no concern for, other human beings. Isolation is the stony soil in which monstrosity takes root.

The self-isolation of the champion of death often becomes evident in his intimate relationships before he gives any political demonstration of his dehumanization. Stalin was a solitary, arrogant, hostile schoolboy, and he maintained his distance from others during his years as a revolutionary. This coldness continued all his life and marked his relationships with his family and his so-called friends. "Friendship is an empty word for him," observed an acquaintance in 1939. "He flung aside and sent to execution such a close friend as Enukidze. . . . He does not even need friends." As for family ties, Stalin never bothered to make the acquaintance of five of his eight grandchildren. He did not respond to gestures of friendship or affection. He ignored his mother's gifts of jam and a blanket that she had made for him. Svetlana observed that "he had created this void around himself with his own hands."

Most manics are constrained by ethics, society, or a basically benign nature from doing grievous harm, but this is not the case with manics who are also tyrants. A former friend of Stalin said, "Scorning people, he considered himself complete master over their life and death." Others were less than nothing to Stalin, except insofar as he found them either useful or threatening. This, too, was the attitude of Napoleon and Hitler. Khrushchev was well aware of the ease with which Stalin killed. "Stalin liked me," he observed. "If he hadn't liked me or if he had felt the slightest suspicion toward me, he could have gotten rid of me anytime he pleased in the same way he got rid of so many people who were undesirable to him."

Because he had no sympathy for any other human being, Stalin's desire for vengeance was without limit. When it was suggested that the opposition must be accommodated in some fashion in order to have peace in the party, Stalin raised his arm in the air and shouted, "They must be crushed!" The Purge, so useful to Stalin in so many ways, also served as an instrument of vengeance against everyone who had ever slighted him. Stalin once remarked, "To choose one's victim, to prepare one's plans minutely, to slake an implacable vengeance, and then to go to bed—there is nothing sweeter in the world."

Not all who are cruel become genocides, but the passion for bloodshed that Stalin showed as a young revolutionary was a sign that he would not hesitate to kill on a mass scale, given the opportunity. He delighted in the suffering of others, and almost choked with laughter at an imitation of one of his victims, Zinoviev, being dragged off to execution. The tyrant wrote obscene comments on petitions for mercy. As the imaginary "Doctors' Plot" was unfolding, Stalin ordered that some of the physicians who served the Kremlin be arrested and forced to confess. Khrushchev related that Stalin ordered the Minister of State Security to "throw the doctors in chains, beat them to a pulp, and grind them into a powder." The dictator yelled, "Beat, beat, and beat yet again." At his orders, torture was made a regular part of interrogation for everyone.

Between 1939 and 1947, Stalin deported more than ten million people plus uncounted millions of Soviet soldiers released from enemy camps. It is impossible to estimate how many survived to reach their destinations and lived long enough to be released during Khrushchev's years of clemency. At Stalin's death there remained 23 million in his camps, most of whom were relatively recent arrivals.

The very immensity of these numbers obscures the individual suffering, the personal tragedies that they tally. Stalin's paranoia turned the Soviet Union into a doom machine. People were arrested simply for being caught at the wrong restaurant table. When a former Vice Premier was seized at an after-theater supper party, everyone with him was taken to prison as well. Three months later, the women were still in their cells, wearing the evening gowns they had worn to the festivities.

THE OLYMPICS OF ANNIHILATION

Hitler and Napoleon both retained in their entourage people whom they knew were damaging them: Goering was incompetent and Talleyrand treacherous. Stalin, on the other hand, killed even those who, like General Yakir, pledged their loyalty in front of the firing squad and died believing in the leader's benevolence.

In their quest for world dominion, Hitler and Napoleon sacrificed millions of their countrymen. Hitler also tried to destroy the Jews, whom he thought of as alien, and other groups and individuals that he considered to be enemies. The Russian dictator differed from the other two in a significant way: he was an enemy of his own people, the worst in its entire history. Stalin directed most of his destructive energies against those who were on his own side: foreign Communists as well as his fellow Russians. The most paranoid of the three tyrants, Stalin never believed in the loyalty of anyone. As Khrushchev attested, "He didn't trust anyone at all." Throughout his years in power, Stalin destroyed his own supporters and persecuted and killed tens of millions of his countrymen. He was the all-time winner of the Olympics of Death.

19

The Modern Tyrant

Economic conditions, political traditions, religion, and history can all contribute to the ascent of a tyrant. But in order to understand and prevent the development of tyranny, one must identify and understand the kind of person who becomes a tyrant, because the tyrant is the keystone sustaining the tyrannical regime. In examining the lives of Napoleon, Hitler, and Stalin to determine if, indeed, there is a special type of human being that becomes a tyrant, we have shown that, despite the vast differences in their backgrounds and the countries they ruled, Napoleon, Hitler, and Stalin were all grandiose manic depressives. All were driven by three forces: unlimited egoism, the compulsion to control everything, and, finally, manic depressive delusions, particularly grandiosity and paranoia.

In the discussion that follows, the behavior described is that of manic depressive tyrants.

BOUNDLESS EGOISM

Bonaparte's, Hitler's, and Stalin's insatiable egoism decreed what version of reality reached their people. They multiplied their names and glorified their images everywhere, then substituted symbolic acts for policies that would benefit their countries.

They created a nation of courtiers who dared not object to anything, who greeted whatever they said or did with enthusiasm, and who worshiped them as though they were gods simply for the privilege of avoiding punishment.

Their concern for the rights and needs of others shrank to the vanishing point while their egos expanded to infinity. Everything and everyone belonged to them, existing only to satisfy their desires, which increased exponentially. Their all-consuming love of self evolved into the delusion that no one else had any importance, that they were everything and the rest of humanity nothing.

WILL AND POWER: THE COMPULSION TO CONTROL EVERYTHING

Tyrannies do not arise by popular demand, but rather by broad deception and the imposition of terror. In the past, religion and traditional attitudes toward the sanctity of the ruler, plus armed force, kept the people in subjugation. Modern tyrants, who, for the most part, no longer have the shields of tradition and religion, buttress themselves with ideologies whose dogma they interpret to suit their own needs. Manic tyrants have no more loyalty to abstract principles than they do to individuals. In some countries, tyrannies have managed to dispense with all ideology except the worship of the leader. Propaganda, political rallies, and mass movements do not bring forth tyrants spontaneously. On the contrary, aspiring tyrants consciously generate these public relations phenomena in their pursuit of power.

In order to shape the thought of his subjects, the tyrant not only seizes control of all information accessible to the public but also turns educational and religious institutions, publications of all kinds, the arts and the sciences into scalpels with which he performs surgery on the minds of his subjects. The gamut of tyranny extends from leaders who meddle occasionally in the lives of their subjects to those who interfere in everything. The limits of control are not set by the desires of the tyrant, for he recognizes no limits. The manic tyrant is constrained only by tradition in traditional autocracies, by the weakness and inefficiency of his bureaucracy, armed forces and police, by the limits of available technology and by the funds that he commands or can borrow.

The most fully developed modern tyrannies, such as those of Nazi Germany and Stalin's Soviet Union, installed constitutions and laws as window dressing. These have become standard equipment since the French Revolution proclaimed "The Rights of Man." However, the legal decor exists in name only, for the tyrant interferes in all legislative and judicial processes. Tyrannies may go through the motions of holding elections but these offer no choice as there is only one legal party and the ruler may select all the candidates if he so wishes. All political opposition, whether by individuals or parties, is illegal.

DELUSIONS OF DIVINITY

The tyrant's excessive egoism merges imperceptibly with grandiosity, as he becomes a captive of delusions common to severe states of mania—he may believe he is divinely selected for some high destiny and possesses powers beyond that of ordinary human beings. The tyrant eventually believes that he has the omniscience, infallibility, and omnipotence of God.

The manic grandiosity of the tyrant has taken many forms over the ages. The oldest traditions, those of hereditary succession, legitimized the ruler as God's choice by birth to wear the crown. Those who ruled by conquest claimed that their martial success was proof God had chosen them. In the Age of Reason, tyrants claimed to have sole knowledge of the laws of statecraft. More recently tyrants have asserted that they were the most accurate interpreters of the pseudoscientific ideologies of German racist fantasies or Marxism. "Nationalist" tyrants designate themselves as the only ones who know what is best for their countries. Religious fanatics present themselves as spokesmen for God. Tyrants find different justifications in different cultures and eras for their persecutions, conquests, and holocausts. The grandiose element is always evident when the tyrant offers no proof of his supposed superiority, but demands his authority be accepted as though it were the will of God.

The modern tyrant may try to appear modest and unassuming, but he either excludes from his government those who would dim his own luster, or else he hides their light under a bushel and jealously denigrates them. Having achieved power, he feels that he is infallible, a genius who already knows everything that is worth knowing. Moreover, the tyrant has no use for people of ability or intelligence, for he believes only in his own. He prefers the company of flatterers who will listen to his monologues. In his arrogance, the tyrant isolates himself from the public and keeps his associates at a distance. He corrupts his own government with his purchases of loyalty, turning gifts into fetters.

The tyrant hates to be contradicted and abominates being shown his errors, to which he remains blind, convinced of his infallibility and perfection. Surrounded by people who constitute an echo chamber, the tyrant hears only what he wants to hear, for the discords of reality are muffled. The tyrant's rages teach his intimidated entourage to hide unpleasant news from him, thus confirming his manic delusions that he is the world's greatest leader. He believes that his country, now become an extension of his own ego, is an emerging Utopia. In peace and war, his rule appears to him a succession of triumphs. He is sure of his divine powers. Having supplanted God, the tyrant is ready to rule the world and improve on the laws of nature.

PARANOIA

The paranoid tyrant assembles his own organization of armed men whose sole function is to serve his consuming need for domination and his insane suspicions. He wants to extinguish all potential for opposition to arise. His secret police scout the population to find more enemies to add to his list, spying on his victims, intimidating them, punishing them, and finally liquidating them. He also turns his suspicions on organizations, professions, and on ethnic and religious groups.

The tyrant recruits his countrymen in his crusade against those he suspects might oppose him. He uses unceasing propaganda to incite mass hysteria and witch hunts, transforming the nation into an army of informers, starting an undeclared civil war of hunters against prey.

His paranoia may infect his country, spreading racism, religious intolerance, and persecution of specific people and groups. Obsessed with vengeance, the tyrant delights in torture and annihilation. Concentration camps and genocide are the final solution, the balm for his burning anxieties.

Tyrants see enemies everywhere within and outside their own borders. Those who can afford it transform their countries into fortress states. Their paranoia turns tyrants into time bombs, set to misinterpret the policies of another head of state as aggression and then order their own forces to attack.

Tyrants, in their monstrous egoism and frenzied fears, are willing to destroy the world rather than submit to defeat.

PREVENTION

Although the Iraqi dictator did not warn the world of his evil intentions by writing about them in a book like *Mein Kampf,* Saddam Hussein's actions gave ample warning of the kind of leader he was. By the time Iraq invaded Iran in September 1980, he had instituted a Stalinist-type purge of both his party and the Iraqi military, had attacked the Kurds with poison gas and deported them, had a long-established secret police, a judicial system based on torture and all the other accoutrements of a modern tyranny.

Had Saddam been recognized then as a murderous, paranoid, grandiose manic, other nations might not have supplied him with such a formidable arsenal. Perhaps, instead, he would have been confined by a coalition powerful enough to keep him harmless. The monstrous dangers of modern tyranny are no longer local phenomena. The greatest threat that tyrants present today is that they can endanger the world if they possess weapons of mass destruction. As both Napoleon and Hitler threatened to bring civilization down in ruins, Saddam Hussein threatened to start World War III rather than relinquish power.

The characteristics of a tyrant, then, are not dependent on a nation's history, degree of development, or specific culture. Tyrannies can arise in any country in which democratic traditions and institutions are either lacking, poorly developed, or weakening. Failing political systems, whether democratic or autocratic, are fertile grounds for the establishment of tyrannies. Nations emerging from colonial rule are especially vulnerable, as was the case with Iraq. Even well-established democracies cannot be considered immune to tyranny. When people are under duress, they may abandon the concepts that guarantee personal liberty.

The greatest obstacle to a saner, safer future lies in the reverence that people have toward those who exercise power over them. Leadership is an essential element in any society, for societies without respect for their leaders either disintegrate or fall prey to more disciplined groups. However, the sanctity of power is a myth humanity can no longer afford. During the American Civil War, a great, benevolent manic-depressive leader spoke of the crisis which threatened the survival of his nation. President Lincoln's message is still in season: "The dogmas of the quiet past are inadequate to the stormy present. The occasion is piled high with difficulty, and we must rise with the occasion. As our case is new, so we must think anew and act anew."

Epilogue

Manic Depression and Contemporary Mass Killers: David Koresh, Jeffrey Dahmer, Jim Jones, and Colin Ferguson

Psychiatry deals with the study, treatment, and prevention of mental disorders. Psychoanalysis, on the other hand, refers to methods of eliciting from patients their past emotional experiences and their role in influencing their current mechanisms by which their pathologic mental state has been produced. The method employs free association, recall, and interpretation of dreams.

Freudian psychoanalytic theory has had an enormous impact on twentieth-century culture, including drama, poetry, fiction, journalism, and even the movie industry. Everywhere psychologizing has influenced how people interpret behavior.

Generations of psychiatrists and other physicians have been indoctrinated into applying psychoanalytic theories to many psychiatric and medical disorders. Psychoanalytic theories have been applied with equal insistence, and equal inappropriateness, to such disorders as asthma, peptic ulcer disease, high blood pressure, ulcerative colitis, and many others.

The dominance of psychoanalysis over psychiatry in the United States would not have come about were it not for the existence in our medical schools of tenure. The power that derives from tenure can, all too easily, transform theory into doctrine.

As a counterpoint to Freud are the pioneering but relatively unknown studies of Emil Kraepelin (1856–1926), a German psychiatrist who developed a classification system for psychiatric disorders. In the sixth edition (1899) of his textbook *Compendium der Psychiatrie,* Kraepelin first made the distinction between manic depressive psychosis and dementia praecox, now called schizophrenia. In *Manic Depressive Insanity and Paranoia,* published in 1921, Kraepelin described and catalogued the cardinal features of manic depressive disorder.

If Krapelin's groundbreaking description of manic depression had had a fraction of the impact of Freud's writings, society would be better equipped to interpret aberrant behavior.

MANIA

Falret and Baillarger (1856), both French psychiatrists, are generally given credit for first describing circular or alternating insanities. Falret insisted that mania and melancholia alternate at regular intervals, and Baillarger that there is a third period of lucidity between these two states. Their classifications were rigid and to a large extent detached from everyday clinical reality. Ultimately Kraepelin (1921) claimed that there were no real differences between a variety of mood states that had been previously observed.

The following is a condensation of Kraepelin's descriptions of mania and depression.

According to Kraepelin, in the slightest form of manic excitement referred to as "hypomania," patients appear livelier and more capable than normal. The patient will often produce witty remarks, puns, startling comparisons, and other products of the imagination. There is a lack of inner unity in the course of ideas; an incapacity to carry out consistently a series of thoughts, to work steadily and logically, and to set in order given ideas; a fickleness of interest; and a sudden and abrupt jumping from one subject to another. In writing and in rhyming a slight "flight of ideas" may make its appearance. That is to say, the patient is easily led away in his narrations to exaggerations and distortions, which arise partly from mistaken perception, but partly also from subsequent misinterpretation of facts and events. There is invariably an exaggerated opinion of the self. The patient often boasts of his performances and capabilities and ridicules the doings of others.

The hypomanic patient cannot be convinced of the real nature of his state. Mood is often exalted and cheerful. The patient is sure of success, feels happy, and sees himself surrounded by pleasant people. There may be a markedly humorous trait but in other hypomanics humor is replaced by great emotional irritability. In this type of hypomania the patient is dissatisfied, intolerant, and fault-finding. He is pretentious and impertinent when he confronts opposition to his wishes and inclinations. Small stresses may bring about violent outbursts of rage. In his fury he may physically attack his family, run amock, set the house on fire, and be verbally abusive. He is impulsive and lacks forethought.

The hypomanic patient is often extremely busy: he has enormous energy and can continue his activity day and night. Work may become very easy as ideas flow. He sleeps little if at all, writes many long letters, keeps a diary and makes numerous phone calls. The patient often dresses in a very ostentatious manner and in company he is often impolite. He often enjoys risqué jokes, carries on boastful conversations, and behaves with unsuitable familiarity toward strangers or his superiors. Many hypomanics become involved in lawsuits which they carry on with great determination.

Hypomanic patients are often sexually excitable, promiscuous, and may develop erotic delusions. They often rationalize their bizarre behavior by claiming medical, marital, or employment problems. Their speech is generally pressured, and they are loquacious.

In the more intense states, referred to as "mania" or "acute mania," patients often develop delusions of grandiosity, divinity, of being descended from a noble family, or possessing great wealth.

DEPRESSION

Kraepelin's description of depression includes the following symptoms: inability to think, chronic fatigue; inattentiveness; impaired memory; slow or labored thinking; calculating incorrectly; making contradictory statements; inability to find words; depersonalization, in which impressions of the external world appear strange and the patient's body feels as if it does not belong to him; inward dejection; gloomy hopelessness; anxiety; restlessness; lack of interest; inability to experience pleasure; humorlessness; dissatisfaction; gloomy thoughts; and lack of self-esteem.

Everything becomes disagreeable to the depressive; everything wearies him —company, music, travel, work. The patient sees only the dark side of things and difficulties; one disappointment and disillusionment follows another. Life seems to be aimless.

In severe delusional depression the subject may have various phobias, including hypochondriacal thoughts and delusions of guilt. Frequently depressed patients lack energy and have difficulty getting up in the morning to get ready for the day. Attending to work and one's personal affairs becomes monumental. In severe delusional depression delusions are often those of persecution, poverty, disease, and paranoia.

Some of Kraepelin's conceptualizations have been open to criticism and modification. However, they form a definitive basis for the diagnosis of mood disorders.

We will now apply Kraepelin's description of manic depression to some of the most infamous mass killers of modern times.

DAVID KORESH

David Koresh, a tyrannical cult leader, took his life and those of eighty-five of his followers in a bloody conflagration in a compound in Waco, Texas, in April 1993. Koresh's megalomaniacal delusions included those of divinity and of being a messiah. He was hypersexual, suicidal, and homicidal. These are textbook symptoms of acute, delusional manic depressive disorder.

A psychiatrist consulted by the FBI insisted that Koresh was an antisocial personality, although his symptoms were only partially consistent with that diagnosis.* The FBI also relied on the advice of experts on hostage situations. No one thought to consult experts on manic depression.

Even if the FBI had been aware that Koresh was a delusional manic depressive, it may not have been able to resolve the conflict. But at least it would have known that, given the nature of manic depressive psychosis, the prospect of settling the conflict by negotiation was negligible. In that light, could ingenious methods have been devised to introduce lithium or an antipsychotic drug into Koresh?

If a deluded, paranoid, tyrannical and violent manic depressive cannot be treated or incarcerated, the only way to stop him may have to be to kill him. Consistent with the lives of many such manic depressives, it was Koresh who ultimately took that step.

JEFFREY DAHMER

In July 1991, Jeffrey Dahmer was arrested in his Milwaukee apartment, in which were found a skeleton, eleven skulls, packages of genitals, and preserved and frozen hearts, muscles, and innards from his seventeen slaughtered victims, all young males.

Prior to commencing his serial killing and cannibalism, Dahmer had been arrested for child molestation and was placed on probation. His probation officer repeatedly wrote in her notes that Dahmer was in a severe depression. Most psychopharmacologists would consider it incomprehensible that she, or her superiors, failed to refer Dahmer for treatment of the depression.

A compulsion is a persistent and irresistible impulse to perform an irrational act. Thus Dahmer had elements of both a mood disorder and a compulsive disorder, an association which is quite common. It is known that many anti-depressants have anticompulsive qualities, and there are reports that anti-

---

*Antisocial personality disorder is characterized by continuous and chronic antisocial behavior in which the rights of others are violated: associated personality traits include impulsiveness, egocentricity, and inability to maintain consistent, responsible functioning at work, at school, or as a parent.

depressants can be effective in remitting pedophilia and other forms of compulsive sexual deviancy, including rape. Antidepressant medication could well have prevented Dahmer from committing his horrendous acts.

JIM JONES

Jim Jones, the evangelical despot, was hypersexual, recurrently depressed, suicidal, and had delusions of paranoia, divinity, and grandeur.

Jones was notorious for his infidelities and had many mistresses. He claimed to masturbate at least thirty times a day. His depression was characterized by suicidal and homicidal impulses; hypochondriasis; self-medication with pain killers, barbiturates and amphetamines; obsession with death and alienation; and suicide attempts. He used antidepressants, taking amitriptyline (Elavil) by injection. He was homicidal from childhood onward and was responsible for the deaths of five investigators, including Congressman Leo Ryan, at an airstrip in Guyana. Ultimately, on November 18, 1978, he ordered over nine hundred of his followers at Jonestown to die by drinking cyanide.

Many of Jones' delusions were both paranoid and depressive. He imagined that people were conspiring against him, and he was obsessed by the prospect of annihilation. Often he expressed fears of the media and government scrutiny.

Jones' manic delusions were chiefly those of divinity and grandeur. He expressed such delusions of divinity as being able to heal the sick and raise the dead. Other manic characteristics he exhibited were domineering behavior and a hunger for unlimited, absolute power.

COLIN FERGUSON

After he had opened fire on evening commuters on the Long Island Railroad, killing five and wounding eighteen, on December 7, 1993, Colin Ferguson was described as a loner with a history of scholastic and occupational failure, rage, racism, and paranoia. Unable to recognize that Ferguson displayed evidence of a psychiatric disorder, the media focused on his upbringing in Jamaica, searching for clues in his environment to explain his motives.

One of the descriptions of Ferguson that appeared in the press stated that he had "meandered through misfortune and failure and perhaps was on the brink of madness." "He had the 'American Dream'; when it fell apart, he looked to blame somebody," his landlord told the press. The landlord added that he thought Ferguson was grandiose.

Ferguson was extremely paranoid. He complained that he was a victim of racial prejudice and rejected state-appointed doctors sent to examine him in an injury case because their surnames sounded ethnic and/or black. In the fall of 1990 Ferguson enrolled at Adelphi University and got into angry confrontations with teachers and students, accusing white students of racism and black activists of being "Uncle Toms." "Black rage will get you," he told a black professor. He talked loudly of violent race wars and revolution. Ferguson once interrupted a lecture by yelling "Kill every white!" In common with other mass murderers, Ferguson compiled a list of complaints and enemies, which was found shortly after his arrest.

Ferguson wrote, phoned, and spoke incessantly to anyone who would listen. At his hearing he could not stop speaking, despite pleas to do so by his attorney and the judge. Ferguson's chatter focused on his complaints that he had not received proper medical care for what seemed to be minor medical or hypochondriacal complaints. All of these symptoms are as characteristic of manic depressive disorder as elevated blood sugar is of diabetes. After the killing ended, Ferguson became extremely contrite, a pattern identical to that recorded of such violent manic depressives as Ivan the Terrible.

Dogmatism and lack of receptiveness to any but the "official" approach may invade any discipline, medical or otherwise. In his book, *Killing the Spirit: Higher Education in America* (1990), Page Smith decries what he sees as "the stubborn refusal of the Academy to acknowledge any truth that does not conform to professional dogma." Similarly in *The Dead Sea Scrolls Deception* (1991), Michael Balgent and Richard Leigh comment: "Those responsible for developing the consensus view have been able to exercise a monopoly over certain crucial sources, regulating the flow of information in a manner that enables its release to serve one's own purposes." This is the phenomenon also explored by Umberto Eco in his novel *The Name of the Rose,* where the monastery and the library within it reflect the medieval church's monopoly of learning, constituting a kind of "closed shop," an exclusive "country club of knowledge" from which all but a select few are banned—a select few prepared to toe the party line. Balgent and Leigh conclude: "To challenge those interpretations is to find one's self labeled at best a crank, at worst a renegade, and an apostate or heretic. Few scholars have the combination of courage, standing, and expertise to issue such a challenge and hold on to their reputation."

References and Bibliography

Abrams, R., and Taylor, M. A. "Unipolar Mania: A Preliminary Report." *Archives of General Psychiatry* 30 (1974): 441–43.

Acheson, Dean. *Sketches From Life: Of Men I Have Known.* New York: Harper and Brothers, 1961.

Akiskal, H. S.; Djenderedjian, A. H.; and Rosenthal, R. H. "Cyclothymic Disorder: Validating Criteria for Inclusion in the Bipolar Affective Group." *American Journal of Psychiatry* 134, no. 11 (1977): 1227–33.

al-Khalil, Samir. *Republic of Fear: The Inside Story of Saddam's Iraq.* New York: Pantheon Books, 1989.

Alliluyeva, Svetlana. *Only One Year.* Trans. Paul Chavichavadze. New York: Harper and Row, 1964.

———. *Twenty Letters to a Friend.* Trans. Priscilla Johnson McMillan. New York: Harper and Row, 1967.

Anderson, Jack, and Clifford, George. *The Anderson Papers.* New York: Random House, 1973.

Antonov-Ovseyenko, Anton. *The Time of Stalin: Portrait of a Tyranny.* Trans. George Saunders. New York: Harper and Row, 1980.

Arendt, Hannah. *The Origins of Totalitarianism.* New York: Meridian Books, 1960.

Baastrup, P. C., and Schou, M. "Lithium as a Prophylactic Agent: Its Effect against Recurrent Depressions and Manic-Depressive Psychosis." *Archives of General Psychiatry* 16 (1967): 162–72.

Balgent, M., and Leigh, R. *The Dead Sea Scrolls Deception.* New York: Summit Books, 1991.

Barber, James David. *The Presidential Character: Predicting Performance in the White House.* Englewood Cliffs, N.J.: Prentice-Hall, Inc., 1972.

Baynes, H. G. *Germany Possessed.* London: Jonathan Cape, 1972.

Belmaker, Robert H., and Van Praag, H. M. *Mania: An Evolving Concept.* New York: S. P. Medical and Scientific Books, 1980.

Berman, Edgar. *Hubert: The Triumph and Tragedy of the Humphrey I Knew.* New York: G. P. Putnam's Sons, 1979.

Bernstein, Carl, and Woodward, Bob. *All The President's Men.* New York: Warner Books, 1975.

Bertrand, Henri-Gratien. *Napoleon at St. Helena.* Trans. Frances Hume. Garden City, N.Y.: Doubleday and Co., Inc., 1952.

Biagli, Enzo. *Svetlana: The Inside Story.* Trans. Timothy Wilson. London: Hodder and Staughton, 1967.

Blake, Robert. *Disraeli.* New York: St. Martin's Press, 1967.

Bonaparte, Napoleon. *"The Corsican": A Diary of Napoleon's Life in His Own Words.* Ed. R. M. Johnston. Boston: Houghton Mifflin Co., Inc., 1910.

————. *Memoirs of Napoleon I.* Ed. F. M. Kircheison and trans. Frederick Collins. New York: Duffield and Co., Inc., 1929.

————. *Memoirs of the Public and Private Life of Napoleon Bonaparte.* 2 vols. London: George Virtue, 1839.

————. *The Mind of Napoleon.* Ed. and trans. J. Christopher Herold. New York: Columbia University Press, 1961.

Bonaparte, Napoleon, and Bonaparte, Josephine. *Confidential Correspondence of the Emperor Napoleon and the Empress Josephine.* Ed. John S. C. Abbott. New York: Mason Brothers, 1860.

Bormann, Martin, and Bormann, Gerda. *The Bormann Letters.* Trans. R. H. Stevens. London: Weidenfeld and Nicolson, 1954.

Bortoli, Georges. *The Death of Stalin.* Trans. Raymond Rosenthal. New York: Praeger Publishers, 1975.

Bourne, Richard. *Political Leaders of Latin America.* New York: Alfred A. Knopf, 1970.

Brain, Lord Russell. "Authors and Psychopaths." *British Medical Journal* 7 (1949): 1427.

————. *Some Reflections on Genius.* New York: Pitman Medical Publishing Co., 1960.

Brzezinski, Zhigniev, and Huntington, Samuel P. *Political Power: USA/USSR.* New York: The Viking Press, 1970.

Brodie, Fawn M. *Richard Nixon: The Shaping of His Character.* New York: W. W. Norton and Co., Inc., 1981.

Bullock, Alan. *Hitler, A Study in Tyranny.* New York: Harper and Row, 1964.

Carlson, G. A.; Davenport, Y. B.; and Jamison, K. "A Comparison of Outcome in Adolescent- and Late-Onset Bipolar Manic-Depressive Illness." *American Journal of Psychiatry* 134, no. 8 (1977): 919–22.

Castelot, Andre. *Napoleon.* Trans. Guy Daniels. New York: Harper and Row, 1971.

Caulaincourt, Duke of Vicenza. *Reflections of Caulaincourt.* London: Henry Colburn, 1838.

————. *With Napoleon in Russia.* Eds. Jean Hanoteau and George Libaire. New York: William Morrow and Co., Inc., 1935.

Clark, Pierce. *Napoleon Self-Destroyed.* New York: Jonathan Cape and Harrison Smith, 1929.

Clarkson, Jesse D. *A History of Russia.* New York: Random House, 1964.

Cohen, Stephen F., ed. *An End to Silence: Uncensored Opinion in the Soviet Union.* Trans. George Saunders. New York: W. W. Norton and Co., Inc., 1982.

Collier, Richard. *Duce!: A Biography of Benito Mussolini.* New York: The Viking Press, 1971.

Conquest, Robert. *The Great Terror: Stalin's Purge of the Thirties.* New York: The Macmillan Co., Inc., 1968.

Constant, Premier Valet de Chambre. *Recollections of the Private Life of Napoleon.* 3 vols. Trans. Walter Clark. New York: Saalfield Publishing Co., 1910.

Crankshaw, Edward. *Khrushchev: A Career.* New York: Viking Press, 1966.

Crassweller, Robert D. *Trujillo: The Life and Times of a Caribbean Dictator.* New York: The Macmillan Co., Inc., 1966.

Cronin, Vincent. *Napoleon Bonaparte: An Intimate Biography.* New York: William Morrow and Co., Inc., 1972.

Crowcroft, Andrew. *The Psychotic: Understanding Madness.* Middlesex, England: Penguin Books, 1975.

Davidson, Eugene. *The Making of Adolf Hitler.* New York: Macmillan Publishing Co., Inc., 1978.

Davies, James C. *Human Nature in Politics: The Dynamics of Political Behavior.* New York: John Willey and Sons, Inc., 1963.

De Bourrienne, Louis Antoine Fauvelet. *Memoirs of Napoleon Bonaparte.* Vol. 3. Ed. R. W. Phipps. New York: Charles Scribner's Sons, 1890.

De Las Cases, Count. *Journal of the Private Life and Conversations of the Emperor Napoleon at St. Helena.* Boston: Wells and Lilly, 1823.

————. *The Military and Political Life, Character, and Anecdotes of Napoleon Bonaparte.* Hartford, 1823.

D'Encausse, Hélène Carrère. *Confiscated Power: How Soviet Russia Really Works.* Trans. George Holoch. New York: Harper and Row, 1982.

De Tocqueville, Alexis. *The Old Regime and the French Revolution.* Trans. Stuart Gilbert. Garden City, N.Y.: Doubleday and Co., Inc., 1955.

Deutscher, Isaac. *Stalin: A Political Biography.* New York: Oxford University Press, 1970.

Dietrich, Otto. *Hitler.* Trans. Richard and Clara Winston. Chicago: Henry Regnery Co., 1955.

Djilas, Milovan. *Conversations With Stalin.* Trans. Michael B. Petrovich. New York: Harcourt, Brace and World, Inc., 1962.

Dollman, Eugene. *The Interpreter: Memoirs of Dr. Eugene Dollman.* Trans. J. Maxwell Brownjohn. London: Hutchinson of London, 1967.

Dorlands Illustrated Medical Dictionary. Philadelphia: W. B. Saunders Co., 1988.

Dornherg, John. *Brezhnev: The Masks of Power.* New York: Basic Books, Inc., 1974.

———. *The New Tsars: Russia under Stalin's Heirs.* Garden City, N.Y.: Doubleday and Co., Inc., 1972.

Ducrest, Madame. *Secret Memoirs of the Court of the Empress Josephine.* 3 vols. Boston: The Grolier Society, 1926.

Dunner, D. L.; Fleiss, J. L.; and Fieve, R. R. "The Course of Development of Mania in Patients With Recurrent Depression." *American Journal of Psychiatry* 133, no. 8 (1976): 905–908.

Dunner, D. L.; Patrick, V.; and Fieve, R. R. "Rapid Cycling in Manic Depressive Patients." *Comprehensive Psychiatry* 18, no. 6 (1977): 561–66.

Ebon, Martin. *Svetlana: The Story of Stalin's Daughter.* New York: The New American Library, 1967.

Eco, U. *The Name of the Rose.* San Diego: Harcourt Brace Jovanovich, 1983.

Fallaci, Oriana. *Interview with History.* Trans. John Shipley. Boston: Houghton Mifflin Co., Inc., 1976.

Farago, Ladislas. *Patton: Ordeal and Triumph.* New York: Dell Publishing Co., Inc., 1970.

Fair, Charles. *From the Jaws of Victory.* New York: Simon and Schuster, 1971.

Fest, Joachim C. *The Face of the Third Reich: Portraits of the Nazi Leadership.* Trans. Michael Bullock. New York: Pantheon Books, 1970.

———. *Hitler.* Trans. Richard and Clara Winston. New York: Harcourt Brace Jovanovich, Inc., 1973.

Fieve, Ronald R. *Moodswing: The Third Revolution in Psychiatry.* New York: Bantam, 1979.

Fishman, Jack, and Bernard, J. Hutton. *The Private Life of Josif Stalin.* London: W. H. Allen, 1962.

Frangos, E.; Athanassesas, G.; Tsitourides, S.; Psilolignos, P.; Robos, A.; Katsanou, N.; and Bulgaris, Ch. "Seasonality of the Episodes of Recurrent Affective Psychoses. Possible Prophylactic Interventions." *Journal of Affective Disorders* 2 (1980): 239–47.

Fromson, Brett Duval. *Running and Fighting: Working in Washington.* New York: Simon and Schuster, 1981.

Gershon, Samuel; and Shopsin, Baron, eds. *Lithium: Its Role in Psychiatric Research and Treatment.* New York:. Plenum Press, 1973.

Gibbs, Montgomery B. *Military Career of Napoleon the Great.* New York: The Saalfield Publishing Co., 1904.

Goebbels, Paul Joseph. *The Goebbels Diaries.* Trans. Louis P. Lochner. Garden City, N.Y.: Doubleday and Co., Inc., 1948.

Goldwin, Robert A.; Stourzh, Gerald; and Zetterbaum, Marvin, eds. *Readings in Russian Foreign Policy.* New York: Oxford University Press, 1959.

Good, Michael I. "Primary Affective Disorder, Aggression, and Criminality: A Review and Clinical Study." *Archives of General Psychiatry* 35 (August 1978).

Goodwin, Frederick K., and Jamison, Kay R. *Manic-Depressive Illness.* New York: Oxford University Press, 1990.

Gourgaud, General Baron. *The St. Helena Journal of General Baron Gourgaud.* Trans. Sidney Gillard and ed. Norman Edwards. London: John Lane the Bodley Head, Ltd., 1932.

Graves, Alonso. *The Eclipse of a Mind.* New York: The Medical Journal Press, 1942.

Guérard, Albert Leon. *Reflections on the Napoleonic Legend.* New York: Charles Scribner's Sons, 1924.

Haffner, Sebastian. *The Meaning of Hitler.* Trans. Ewald Osers. New York: Macmillan Publishing Co., Inc., 1979.

Halberstam, David. *The Best and the Brightest.* New York: Fawcett Crest Books, 1972.

Haldeman, H. R., with Di Mona, Joseph. *The Ends of Power.* New York: Dell Publishing Co., Inc., 1978.

Hanfstaengl, Ernst. *Unheard Witness.* New York: J. B. Lippincott, 1957.

Hassanyeh, F., and Davison, K. "Bipolar Affective Psychosis With Onset before Age 16 Years: Report of 10 Cases." *British Journal of Psychiatry* 137 (1980): 530–39.

Helge, Lundholm. *The Manic-Depressive Psychosis.* Durham, N.C.: Duke University Press, 1931.

Hershman, D. Jablow, and Lieb, Julian. *The Key to Genius: Manic-Depression and the Creative Life.* Buffalo, N.Y.: Prometheus Books, 1988.

Heston, Leonard L., and Heston, Renate. *The Medical Casebook of Adolf Hitler.* New York: Stein and Day, 1979.

Hingley, Ronald. *Joseph Stalin: Man and Legend.* New York: McGraw-Hill Book Co., 1974.

Hitler, Adolf. *Hitler's Table Talk.* Trans. Norman Cameron and R. H. Stevens. London: Wiedenfeld and Nicolson, 1973.

———. *Mein Kampf.* Trans. Ralph Manheim. Boston: Houghton Mifflin Co., Inc., 1971.

———. *Secret Conversations With Hitler: The Two Newly Discovered 1931 Interviews.* Ed. Edouard Calic. New York: The John Day Co., 1971.

Hughes, Emmet John. *The Ordeal of Power: A Political Memoir of the Eisenhower Years.* New York: Dell Publishing Co., Inc., 1962.

Hyde, H. Montgomery. *Stalin: The History of a Dictator.* London: Rupert Hart-Davis Ltd., 1971.

Infield, Glenn B. *Eva and Adolf.* New York: Grosset and Dunlap, 1974.

Kalb, Marvin, and Kalb, Bernard. *Kissinger.* Boston: Little, Brown and Co., Inc., 1974.

Kaplan, Bert, ed. *The Inner World of Mental Illness.* New York: Harer and Row, 1964.

Kaplan, Fred. *The Wizards of Armageddon.* New York: Simon and Schuster, 1983.

Kearns, Doris. *Lyndon Johnson and the American Dream.* New York: Harper and Row, 1976.

Khrushchev, Nikita Sergeyevich. *Khrushchev Remembers.* Trans. Strobe Talbott. Boston: Little, Brown and Co., Inc., 1970.

———. *Khrushchev Remembers: The Last Testament.* Trans. and ed. Strobe Talbott. Boston: Little, Brown and Co., 1974.

———. *The Secret Speech.* Trans. Tamara Deutscher. New York: Spokesman Books, 1976.

Koslow, Jules. *Ivan the Terrible.* New York: Hill and Wang, 1961.

Kraepelin, Emil. *Manic-Depressive Insanity and Paranoia.* Trans. R. Mary Barclay and ed. George M. Robertson. Edinburgh: F. and S. Livingstone, 1921. Reprint New York: Arno Press, 1976.

Krauthammer, C., and Klerman, G. L. "Secondary Mania. Manic Symptoms Associated With Antecedent Physical Illness or Drugs." *Archives of General Psychiatry* 35 (1978): 1333–39.

Krock, Arthur. *The Consent of the Governed and Other Deceits.* Boston: Little, Brown and Co., Inc., 1971.

Kronfol, Z.; Silva, J., Jr.; Greden, J.; Dembinski, S.; Gardener, R.; and Carroll, B.. "Impaired Lymphocyte Function in Depressive Illness." *Life Sciences* 33 (1983): 241–47.

Kubizek, August. *The Young Hitler I Knew.* Trans. E. V. Anderson. Boston: Houghton Mifflin Co., 1955.

Kurzman, Dan. *Ben-Gurion: Prophet of Fire.* New York: Simon and Schuster, 1983.

Kvemba, Henry. *A State of Blood: The Inside Story of Idi Amin.* New York: Grosset and Dunlap, 1977.

Lacayo, R. "In the Grip of a Psychopath." *Time,* May 3, 1993, pp. 34–35.

Lacouture, Jean. *The Demigods: Charismatic Leadership in the Third World.* Trans. Patricia Wolf. New York: Alfred A. Knopf, 1970.

———. *Nasser: A Biography.* Trans. Daniel Hofstadter. New York: Alfred A. Knopf, 1973.

Lamb, David. *The Africans.* New York: Random House, 1982.

Langer, Walter C. *The Mind of Adolf Hitler.* New York: Basic Books, Inc., 1972.

Lasky, Victor. *JFK: The Man and the Myth.* New York: Dell Publishing Co., Inc., 1977.

Leiden, Carl, and Schmitt, Karl M. *The Politics of Violence: Revolution in the Modern World.* Englewood Cliffs, N.J.: Prentice-Hall, Inc., 1968.

Leonhard, Wolfgang. *Child of the Revolution.* Chicago: Henry Regnery Co., 1958.

Levy, Arthur. *The Private Life of Napoleon.* Trans. Stephen Louis Simeon. London: Richard Bentley and Son, 1894.

Lieb, J. *A Medical Solution to the Health Care Crisis.* St. Louis, Mo.: Warren H. Green, 1993.

————. "Schizophrenia or Manic-Depression?" *The Lancet* 2 (1983): 918.

Lipson, E. *Europe in the 19th Century.* New York: Collier Books, 1966.

Loranger, A. W., and Levine, P. M. "Age at Onset of Bipolar Affective Illness." *Archives of General Psychiatry* 35 (1978): 1345–48.

Ludwic, Emil. *Napoleon.* Trans. Eden and Cedar Paul. New York: Boni and Liveright, 1926.

Lurie, Leonard. *Party Politics: Why We have Poor Presidents.* New York: Stein and Day, 1980.

McCormick, R. A.; Russo, A. M.; Ramirez, L. F.; et al. "Affective Disorders among Pathological Gamblers Seeking Treatment." *American Journal of Psychiatry* 141, no. 2 (1984): 215–18.

McPherson, Harry. *A Political Education.* Boston: Little, Brown and Co., Inc., 1972.

MacPherson, Myra. *The Power Lovers: An Intimate Look at Politicians and Their Marriages.* New York: G. P. Putnam's Sons, 1975.

Magnus, Philip. *Gladstone: A Biography.* New York: E. P. Dutton and Co., Inc., 1964.

Manchester, William. *American Caesar: Douglas MacArthur.* Boston: Little, Brown and Co., Inc., 1978.

————. *The Arms of Krupp.* Boston: Little, Brown and Co., Inc., 1968.

Marie-Louise, Empress. *The Private Diaries of Empress Marie-Louise.* Ed. Frédéric Masson. D. Appleton and Co., 1922.

Massie, Robert K. *Peter The Great: His Life and World.* New York: Alfred A. Knopf, 1980.

Maurois, André. *A History of France.* Trans. Henry L. Binsse. New York: Farrar, Strouse and Cudahy, 1956.

Medvedev, Roy. *Khrushchev.* Trans. Brian Pearce. Garden City, N.Y.: Anchor Press/Doubleday, 1983.

————. *Let History Judge: The Origins and Consequences of Stalinism.* Trans. Coleen Taylor and eds. David Joravsky and Georges Haupt. New York: Random House, 1971.

Medvedev, Zhores. *Andropov.* New York: W. W. Norton and Co., Inc., 1983.

Mendels, Joseph. *Concepts of Depression.* New York: John Wiley and Sons, Inc., 1970.

Méneval, Baron Claude-François de. *Memoirs Illustrating the History of*

Napoleon I From 1802 to 1815. Trans. Robert H. Sherard. New York: D. Appleton and Co., 1984.

Meser, Werner, *Hitler: Legend, Myth and Reality.* Trans. Peter and Betty Ross. New York: Harper and Row, 1975.

Miller, Judith, and Mylroie, Laurie. *Saddam Hussein and the Crisis in the Gulf.* New York: Times Books, 1990.

Miller, William "Fishbait," and Leighton, Frances Patty. *Fishbait: The Memoirs of the Congressional Doorkeeper.* Englewood Cliffs, N.J.: Prentice-Hall, Inc., 1977.

Moraes, Dom. *Indira Gandhi.* Boston: Little, Brown and Co., Inc., 1980.

Morrison, J. R. "Bipolar Affective Disorder and Alcoholism." *American Journal of Psychiatry* 131, no. 10 (1974): 1130–33.

Moseley, Philip E. *The Kremlin and World Politics: Studies in Soviet Policy and Action.* New York: Vintage Books, 1960.

Mukherjee, S.; Shukla, S.; Woodle, J.; et al. "Misdiagnosis of Schizophrenia in Bipolar Patients: A Multiethnic Comparison." *American Journal of Psychiatry* 140, no. 12 (1983): 1571–74.

Norman, Barbara. *Napoleon and Talleyrand: The Last Two Weeks.* New York: Stein and Day, 1976.

Nugent, John Peer. *Call Africa 999.* New York: Coward-McCann, Inc., 1965.

Oldenberg, Zoe. *Catherine the Great.* Trans. Anne Carter. New York: Random House, 1965.

Paykel, E. S., ed. *Handbook of Affective Disorders.* New York: The Guilford Press, 1982.

Payne, Robert. *Great Man: A Portrait of Winston Churchill.* New York: Coward, McCann and Geoghegan, 1974.

———. *The Life and Death of Adolf Hitler.* New York: Popular Library, 1973.

———. *The Life and Death of Mahatma Gandhi.* New York: E. P. Dutton and Co., Inc., 1969.

———. *The Rise and Fall of Stalin.* New York: Simon and Schuster, 1965.

Pearson, Drew, and Anderson, Jack. *The Case against Congress.* New York: Simon and Schuster, 1968.

Perlmutter, Amos. *Modern Authoritarianism: A Comparative Institutional Analysis.* New Haven: Yale University Press, 1981.

Perris, C. "The Separation of Bipolar (Manic-Depressive) from Unipolar Recurrent Depressive Psychoses." *Behavioral Neuropsychiatry* 1, no. 8 (1969): 17–24.

Polmar, Norman, and Allen, Thomas B. *Rickover.* New York: Simon and Schuster, 1982.

Pope, H. G., and Lipinski, J. F. "Diagnosis of Schizophrenia and Manic-Depressive Illness." *Archives of General Psychiatry* 35 (1978): 811–28.

Rauschning, Hermann. *Hitler Speaks.* London: Eyre and Spottiswoode, 1940.

Reeves, Thomas C. *The Life and Times of Joe McCarthy: A Biography.* New York: Stein and Day, 1982.

Reich, L. H.; Davies, R. K.; and Himmelhoch, J. M. "Excessive Use of Alcohol in Manic-Depressive Illness." *American Journal of Psychiatry* 131, no. 1 (1974): 83–86.

Riedel, Richard Langham. *Halls of the Mighty: My 42 Years at the Senate.* Washington, D.C.: Robert B. Luce, Inc., 1969.

Rigby, T. H. *Stalin.* Englewood Cliffs, N.J.: Prentice-Hall, Inc., 1966.

Robinson, Logan. *An American in Leningrad.* New York: W. W. Norton and Co., Inc., 1982.

Rose, J. Holland. *The Personality of Napoleon.* New York: G.P. Putnam's Sons, 1912.

Rosenberg, Alfred. *Memoirs of Alfred Rosenberg.* Trans. Eric Posselt. Chicago: Ziff-Davis Publishing Co., 1949.

Ross, Michael. *The Reluctant King: Joseph Bonaparte.* New York: Mason/ Charter, 1977.

Russell, Francis. *The President Makers: From Mark Hanna to Joseph P. Kennedy.* Boston: Little, Brown and Co., Inc., 1976.

Saffire, William. *Before The Fall: An Inside View of the Pre-Watergate White House.* New York: Ballantine Books, 1977.

Savant, Jean. *Napoleon in His Time.* Trans. Katherine John. New York: Thomas Nelson and Sons, 1958.

St. Denis, Louis Étienne. *Napoleon from the Tuileries to St. Helena.* Trans. Frank Hunter Potter. New York: Harper and Brothers, 1922.

Schmidt, Paul. *Hitler's Interpreter.* Ed. R. H. C. Steed. New York: Macmillan Co., Inc., 1951.

Schoenbrun, David. *The 3 Lives of Charles de Gaulle: A Biography.* New York: Atheneum, 1966.

Schou, M. "Artistic Productivity and Lithium Prophylaxis in Manic-Depressive Illness." *British Journal of Psychyatry* 135 (1979): 97–103.

Schram, Stuart. *Mao Tse-Tung.* New York: Simon and Schuster, 1966.

Seaton, Albert. *Stalin as Warlord.* London: B. T. Batsford, 1976.

Shanor, Donald R. *The Soviet Triangle.* New York: St. Martin's Press, 1980.

Shirer, William L. *The Rise and Fall of the Third Reich.* New York: Simon and Schuster, 1960.

Shogan, Robert. *None of the Above: Why Presidents Fail and What Can Be Done about It.* New York: New American Library, 1982.

Shopsin, Baron. *Manic Illness.* New York: Raven Press, 1979.

Sidey, Hugh. *A Very Personal Presidency: Lyndon Johnson in the White House.* New York: Atheneum, 1968.

Simon, Paul. *The Glass House: Politics and Morality in the Nation's Capital.* New York: Continuum, 1984.

Simon, W. M. *Germany: A Brief History.* New York:. Random House, 1966.

Sims, Konstantin M. *USSR: The Corrupt Society.* Trans. Jacqueline Edwards and Mitchell Schneider. New York: Simon and Schuster, 1983.

Smith, Hedrick. *The Russians.* New York: Quadrangle/The New York Times Book Co., 1976.

Smith, P. *Killing the Spirit: Higher Education in America.* New York: Viking, 1990.

Snow, Edgar. *The Long Revolution.* New York: Random House, 1972.

Sokoloff, Boris. *Napoleon: A Doctor's Biography.* New York: Prentice-Hall, Inc., 1937.

Souvarine, Boris. *Stalin: A Critical Survey of Bolshevism.* New York: Longmans, Green and Co., 1939.

Speer, Albert. *Inside the Third Reich.* Trans. Richard and Clara Winston. New York: Macmillan Publishing Co., Inc., 1970.

Stein, George H., ed. *Hitler.* Englewood Cliffs, N.J.: Prentice-Hall, Inc., 1968.

Strasser, Otto. *Hitler and I.* Trans. Gwenda David and Eric Mosbacher. Boston: Houghton Mifflin Co., 1940.

Strout, Richard L. *TRB: Views and Perspectives on the Presidency.* New York: Macmillan Publishing Co., Inc., 1979.

Suvorov, Victor. *Inside the Soviet Army.* New York: Macmillan Publishing Co., Inc., 1982.

Symonds, R. L., and Williams, P. "Seasonal Variation in the Incidence of Mania." *British Journal of Psychiatry* 129 (1976): 45–48.

Szulc, Tad. *Twilight of the Tyrants.* New York: Henry Holt and Co., 1959.

Tarlé, Eugene. *Bonaparte.* Trans. John Cournos. New York: Knight Publications, 1937.

Taylor, A. J. P. *Bismark: The Man and the Statesman.* New York: Random House, 1967.

Toland, John. *Adolf Hitler.* Garden City, N.Y.: Doubleday and Co., Inc., 1976.

Toufexis, A. "A Mass Murderer's Journey toward Madness." *Time,* December 20, 1993, p. 25.

Trotsky, Leon. *Stalin: An Appraisal of the Man and His Influence.* Ed. and trans. Charles Malamuth. New York: Stein and Day, 1967.

Tucker, Robert C. *Stalin as a Revolutionary: A Study in History and Personality.* New York: W. W. Norton and Co., Inc., 1973.

Ulam, Adam B. *Expansionism and Coexistence: The History of Soviet Foreign Policy, 1917–1967.* New York: Frederick A. Praeger, 1968.

———. *Stalin: The Man and His Era.* New York: Viking Press, 1973.

U'Ren, R. "Schizophrenia or Manic-Depression?" *The Lancet* 2 (1983): 918.

Valenti, Jack. *A Very Human President.* New York: W. W. Norton and Co., Inc., 1975.

Valeriani, Richard. *Travels With Henry.* New York: Berkley Books, 1979.

Vernadsky, George. *A History of Russia.* New Haven: Yale University Press, 1961.

Von Papen, Franz. *Memoirs.* Trans. Brian Connell. New York: E. P. Dutton and Co., Inc., 1953.

Von Ribbentrop, Joachim. *The Ribbentrop Memoirs.* Trans. Oliver Watson. London: Weidenfeld and Nicolson, 1954.

Waite, Robert G. L. *The Psychopathic God: Adolf Hitler.* New York: Basic Books, Inc., 1977.

Waugh, Elizabeth. *Simon Bolivar: A Story of Courage.* New York: The Macmillan Co., Inc., 1943.

Weber, Max. *The Theory of Social and Economic Organization.* Trans. A. M. Henderson and Talcott Parsons. New York: The Free Press, 1964.

Weider, Ben, and Hapgood, David. *The Murder of Napoleon.* New York: Congdon and Lattes, Inc., 1982.

Weissman, Myrna M.; Fox, Karen; and Klerman, Gerald L. "Hostility and Depression Associated with Suicide Attempts." *American Journal of Psychiatry* 130 (April 1973): 4.

Weissman, Myrna M., and Paykel, Eugene S. *The Depressed Woman: A Study of Social Relationships.* Chicago. The University of Chicago Press, 1974.

White, Theodore H. *Breach of Faith: The Fall of Richard Nixon.* New York: Atheneum Publishers, 1975.

————. *The Making of the President 1964.* New York: The New American Library, Inc., 1965.

Wicker, Tom. *JFK and LBJ: The Influence of Personality upon Politics.* New York: Penguin Books, 1976.

Williams, T. Harry. *Huey Long: A Biography.* New York: Alfred A. Knopf, 1969.

Wilson, Dick. *The People's Emperor: Mao. A Biography of Mao Tse-Tung.* Garden City, N.Y.: Doubleday and Co., Inc., 1980.

Winoker, George; Clayton, Paula J.; and Reich, Theodore. *Manic Depressive Illness.* St. Louis: C. V. Mosby, 1969.

Wolfe, Bertram. *Three Who Made a Revolution: A Biographical History.* Boston: Beacon Press, 1948.

Wolpert, Edward A., ed. *Manic-Depressive Illness: History of a Syndrome.* New York: International Universities Press, Inc., 1977.

Woodward, Bob, and Bernstein, Carl. *The Final Days.* New York: Avon Books, 1977.

Wright, L. "Orphans of Jonestown." *The New Yorker,* November 22, 1993, pp. 66–89.

Yao Ming-le. *The Conspiracy and Death of Lin Biao.* New York: Alfred A. Knopf, 1983.